MY ANIMAL KINGDOM, ONE BY ONE

I think I could turn and live with animals,
    they are so placid and self-contain'd,
I stand and look at them long and long.
They do not sweat and whine about their condition,
They do not lie awake in the dark and weep
    for their sins,
They do not make me sick discussing their duty to God,
Not one is dissatisfied, not one is demented
    with the mania of owning things,
Not one kneels to another, nor to his kind
    that lived thousands of years ago,
Not one is respectable or unhappy over the
    whole earth.

Walt Whitman, *Song of Myself*

MY
ANIMAL
KINGDOM,
ONE BY ONE

David Taylor

STEIN AND DAY/*Publishers*/New York

First published in the United States of America in 1984
Copyright © 1984 by David Taylor
All rights reserved, Stein and Day, Incorporated
Printed in the United States of America
STEIN AND DAY / *Publishers*
Scarborough House
Briarcliff Manor, N.Y. 10510
Originally published in England as *The Wandering Whale*.

Library of Congress Cataloging in Publication Data

Taylor, David, 1934-
    My animal kingdom, one by one.

    1. Taylor, David, 1934-   2. Veterinarians—
England—Biography. 3. Zoo animals—Diseases. 4. Wild-
life diseases. 1. Title.
SF613.T38A357 1984   636.089′092′4 [B]   83-40581
ISBN 0-8128-2963-8

To my very good compañero,
Robert Bennett

Contents

1 The Wandering Whale

The boy in the rowing boat went white as a sheet and slipped backwards off his seat. He collided with the two plastic buckets standing in the bottom of the boat and their contents, an evening's haul of crabs, spilled out and began to leg it for cover. The cause of the boy's alarm was a large blob of opaque jelly that had shot suddenly over the side of the boat and landed, warm and slimy, on his face. He heard a short, deep, rushing noise close by and felt something push the little craft from underneath, making it lurch suddenly in the still water. His reel and line, forsaken, spiralled down into the murky brown sea. In a panic of disquiet he pawed at the sticky ooze sliding down his cheek with one hand, grabbed an oar with the other and looked over the side. A foot away, a black curved fin was slicing through the surface of the sea. Beneath the fin, slowly rising, was a long dark shadow, longer by far than the little rowing boat. Jaws! Shark attack! The boy's scalp began to creep eerily. He felt instantly sick, a stomach-screwing mixture of apprehension, fear and excitement. A sea-monster within spitting distance – he trembled violently. Was it aware of his presence? Had it come to him? *For* him? Unnoticed, the sweat-beads swelled on his forehead, glinting in the soft orange light.

The shadow darkened still further, turned charcoal-grey and emerged, a glistening five-metre-long body. Near one end a vent opened with a soft, explosive sound and there was another brief rush of air accompanied by a bubbling of mucus.

1

'Bloody heck!' shouted the boy – but there was nobody to hear him except the big, dying whale lying alongside.

They were about two hundred yards offshore, at high tide on a lonely bit of coast to the north of Grange-over-Sands. In the distance the fells of the Lake District glowed from a sun that at sea level had already dissolved into the horizon. Closer to were fields with dark dry-stone walls, clumps of hawthorn and gorse and wiry grass. Gulls swirled across the land like paper litter. At the sea-edge the fields ended with a thin crust of shingle fringed with wavelets, below which the beach shelved gently away, first the sand and then mud that would be exposed for miles out at low tide. This was the haunt of flocks of dunlins and little stints, busy and gregarious as city sparrows, and the shallow sea here was rich in the shrimps and hydrobia snails that such birds relish. But it wasn't regular whale country.

The boy now realised what he was looking at, though he had never heard of whales being reported in these waters, let alone seen one. With his initial fright turning to high elation, he watched the dark grey body move slowly onwards, submerging every few seconds and then surfacing to blow a feeble breath. He didn't know, as he watched the whale sail towards the shore, that this faster-than-normal respiration and the discharge being thrown out of the blow hole were signs of mortal illness. His astonishment was quickly tinged by concern, however, for on that course the leviathan was bound to run aground and beach itself. 'Hey, whoah up!' he bawled and, setting his oars firmly, he began to swing the boat round and to follow the whale. 'Please, God, turn the poor great beast away before it runs aground.' He overtook it easily, shipped the oars, leaned over the side and began to splash water in front of the approaching animal with his hands. 'Go back you daft ha'porth – go on, bugger off!' He splashed violently till the tip of the whale's snout was just below him. It took not a blind bit of notice and passed him by again.

Next the boy used an oar to cause a commotion in the water,

pulling the boat round until it was squarely between whale and beach. With all his strength he whacked the wooden blade on the water. Curtains of spray glinted in the golden light and the little boat rocked violently. The whale slipped smoothly beneath the boy and rose again beyond him. He could see the lazy rise and fall of its tail as it travelled the last few feet to the slope of sand. With a gentle crunch the whale touched the beach, its tail flukes flailed wildly three or four times above the water surface and it slewed round. Falling onto its side, the whale gave a great sigh and lay, as if in deep contentment, with the upper two-thirds of its body exposed on the sand.

The boy sat in his boat and stared in terrible fascination. The only sounds were the lapping of water against the whale's belly and the sad cry of curlew on the moors beyond. He had witnessed the strange and mysterious landfall of a creature that rightly belonged to the deep ocean: a seven-ton, leg-less, air-breathing mammal had stranded itself, apparently wilfully, on the north Lancashire coast. The boy pulled hard for the beach, his heart galloping. He had to tell his dad!

Dad, a farmer, was dipping sheep in pens a mile away. When his panting, shouting, red-faced son appeared, he waited until the boy was able to gasp out the story and then trotted off to a telephone box down on the Meathop Road. He rang the local police sergeant and set in motion a chain of communication. The sergeant phoned the RSPCA inspector and the coast-guard. The coastguard, going by the book, phoned the Natural History Museum (Whales Section), which was closed because it was a Sunday evening. He didn't try phoning the Queen at Buckingham Palace, even though the whale lying above the low-water mark technically belonged to her. Stranded whales and dolphins being the Sovereign's property, it is odd how rarely the Duke of Edinburgh or Captain Mark Phillips comes dashing out to claim these windfalls for the family. Perhaps one day if they build an oceanarium in Sandringham. . . ? The RSPCA inspector phoned headquarters. And headquarters phoned my friend, Reg Bloom in Clacton-on-Sea, organiser of the Whale Rescue Unit.

When the radio telephone started to bleep the alarm I was near Bristol, heading home after visiting Cardiff to lance a boil on a circus elephant. I turned round and took the M5 north. Two and a half hours and one speeding ticket later, I was on the beach by the hamlet of Lindale. The tide was now well out and the whale lay like a giant salamander far from the water's edge in the light of a propane lamp. It had been sensibly draped in wet seaweed and the boy's father was sprinkling it with water he had brought down in two milk churns on the back of a tractor. The identification of the animal was easy. Charcoal-grey with a slightly paler abdomen, a round high forehead like the bows of a nuclear submarine, long sickle-shaped flippers and a long low dorsal – it was an Atlantic pilot whale, sometimes called a caa'ing whale or Atlantic black fish, an old female. Her teeth were yellow and most were worn level with the gums, but she could still eat: she had vomited several hundred small squid just before I arrived.

Walking round her, I listened to the bubbling breathing. Her breath smelled bad and she was now blowing out flecks of dark blood with the mucus. The blow hole stayed open far too long when she breathed. I could look down into the nostrils and see dark liquid in the upper diverticulae. These anatomical crevices were designed to catch spray and spume inhaled when the whale rolled in the great ocean breakers, not blood. There was no doubt about it: whatever the reason for her stranding, she was now dying unpleasantly. Trying to refloat her would be both futile and cruel.

The group of men gathered round and I explained the position. 'No point in heroics. The outlook's sad but certain. Our job now is to give her a peaceful end.'

'But couldn't we just try refloating it?' The boy who had first met the pilot whale sounded close to tears.

'We could refloat it, but it will undoubtedly die in the process

4

or beach again quickly. I'm against pulling it two miles out just to let it die a miserable death soon after.'

The whale's breathing was becoming more laboured and difficult by the minute. With no water to support its great chest, it was literally being suffocated by its own weight. 'It's best put to sleep,' said the police sergeant, 'but how do you do that, Doctor?'

Euthanasia is a necessary and important part of veterinary work. One of the advantages of wildlife medicine is that far less often than my general practice colleagues, particularly those who work with small animals, do I have to kill animals. With the vast majority of my patients we fight on to the bitter end, if necessary neutralising pain or discomfort with powerful analgesics and sedatives, but kill I must from time to time.

To euthanase this whale correctly would make my long journey to the north more than worthwhile. Not many people have any idea of how to go about the sad task and bizarre things have happened. The vet, RSPCA inspector or policeman faced with one of the twenty to thirty whales stranded on average each year round the British coasts is faced with problems of anatomy if euthanasia is preferred to refloating. Shoot it – yes, but where? A whale possesses a large, round forehead in front of the blow hole, and it looks as if the brain should lie somewhere in there. Not a bit of it. Everything in front of the blow hole is fat, in the case of many species a semi-liquid fat that acts as a sound lens for focusing the sonar beam. I had seen cases where well-meaning marksmen had shot the whale there, 'in the head'. Useless. Even knowing where the brain is, deep in such an enormous creature, is of little use unless one has a powerful weapon that can penetrate dense blubber and bone. A .22 rifle or most makes of pistol other than a magnum special are useless. Other methods? I had known one horrific case where an individual had tried to saw the head off a living whale, another where water had been poured down a blow hole. It was to help stop such barbarity that Andrew Greenwood, my partner, and I published a short note in the

5

Veterinary Record, explaining how to go about it. We had discovered a drug which could be given even through a short needle in tiny amounts anywhere on a whale's body and produce rapid, painless death. It is the powerful Immobilon, which is widely used for anaesthesia of horses, dogs and also many species of zoo animals. A morphine derivative, it is a first-class narcotic for veterinary use but some animals are highly sensitive to it. These include cats, primates (including man), elephants, tapirs – and whales. Incredibly tiny doses knock out these species and overdoses bring sure and pain-free release.

My black bag contained as ever a bottle of Immobilon. I drew a teaspoonful into a syringe and bent over the whale. The drug would take only a few minutes if given intramuscularly but I decided to end its misery even faster. With the police sergeant holding the lamp close, I found a tail fluke vein and slipped in the lethal liquid. It took about thirty seconds for the drug to travel up to the heart, out to the lungs, back to the heart again and finally to the brain. When it did, the whale simply stopped breathing and was gone. 'I'll do an autopsy in the morning,' I said. 'Maybe we'll find out then why this old lady came ashore.'

As we moved away, the lamplight fell momentarily upon the face of the young boy, who had been standing a little way off. I glimpsed the glistening eyes and mouth twisted in grief. It was *his* whale.

Next day it was raining cats and dogs and aardvarks. A strong wind blew in from the sea as I stood over the corpse of the pilot whale, naked except for my underpants (perfect attire for al fresco whale dissection, I have found – it stops Hanne, my wife, having a fit when I return with gore-sodden clothes). The farmer had promised me a bath. Veterinary work is not what many fond mums seem to think it is when they tell me what a marvellous vet their little Clifford or Ermintrude would make – 'Heartbroken when he lost his pet mouse.' Or 'She's dotty about the pony club.' Love of the science of disease is what it's really all about. Guts and blood and pain and death are my familiars. Whale autopsies are pathology writ large and uncomfortable, and usually without benefit of heated post mortem room, showers, block and tackle or white-coated assistants. It is back-breaking work, exposed to the elements and often odorous, since whales are sometimes several days dead when first discovered. Saws and meat hooks are more valuable than scalpels and forceps and it is sometimes necessary actually to climb inside the cold cadaver to explore the wonders of these most mysterious of beasts.

Not for the squeamish, you say? The fascination of the work, of getting to grips with the fundamental processes of life and death in organisms more intricate and more perfect than any machine, obliterates such considerations. By the end of the morning's dissection I had found two things wrong with the old pilot whale: a terminal pneumonia and bronchitis and, what intrigued me more, both inner ears packed with writhing masses of small black worms. On its last run, I was sure, the whale had been deaf as a post.

The Lindale whale raised again the long-standing question of why whales strand themselves. There are several possible explanations: illness, where an animal might crave some support to keep its blow hole above water; panic caused by killer whale attack; violent storms or underwater volcanic eruptions; disorientation due to faults in the sonar system. This last possibility was of interest in the present case because so many strandings of whales have occurred, as at Lindale, on gently sloping, sandy coasts. Perhaps the echo-location signals are confused by this sort of geography. Again, the ear-worms common in cetaceans (i.e. whales, porpoises and the like) would destroy an animal's capacity to receive and home in on its own sonar beam. I tended strongly toward the worm damage explanation in this case.

The most modern theory, particularly for mass strandings, is that whales, which once lived on land and then gradually moved out to sea, will in times of stress return for refuge to their ancestral 'safehouse', the land, just as their forbears

7

would have done long ago at the stage of evolution when they were halfway between being truly terrestrial and truly aquatic. They respond in other words to an instinctive impulse when times are hard.

This idea has never really grabbed me, but there is another hypothesis which is also applicable to the spectacular beaching of groups of whales: ancient migration routes. Perhaps, it is said, the animals follow, lemming-like, some primeval path across the oceans now blocked by the ever-shifting land masses. It is an appealing theory and, about a year after the local environmental health department had disposed of the remains of Lindale's old pilot whale, I had the opportunity to be present at a unique and fortuitous experiment to explore this possibility. If the long-lost migration route theory is correct, all that is wrong for the whales is that a chunk of land – Great Britain or Africa or Australia, say, – has impertinently obstructed their right of way. Move it and they would, no doubt, doff their caps and continue politely on their way. Unfortunately it is difficult to give land masses the old heave-ho just because Moby Dick is toddling from A to B. But, as the saying goes, if Mohammed won't go to the mountain. . . .

I heard about it shortly after it occurred. A school of false killer whales, thirty-four in all, had stranded themselves on the sandy shore near Daytona Beach on the eastern coast of the Florida Keys. I took the next flight down to Miami. Various agencies, from the State Department of Fish and Game through Greenpeace to the local humane society, were involved in trying to refloat the whales and set them off again for the open sea. Friends of mine, vets at the Miami Seaquarium, had a more exciting idea. They planned to take one or two whales overland to St Petersburg on Florida's western coast. If the whales were released there, then maybe, with the Florida Keys 'removed', they would continue making a bee-line for wherever they were going instead of stubbornly doing a U-turn and returning to the land as stranded whales so often will.

That would have proved the migration path theory, but it didn't work out. After much effort in packing and shipping the whales across the Keys and re-launching them, they invariably charged back onto the beach again with infuriating persistence, as if they had an overwhelming death wish. They behaved no more sensibly than their fellows pushed out to sea on the east coast. A few did see the light and go, but many died on shore and we found ear-worms in all of them at post mortem. I wonder if we will ever find the answer to this age-old mystery.

As for me, I adore seeing and touching whales but not like this – washed-up kings of the sea, for all their glory as spent and forlorn as pieces of driftwood. The dry land of this earth is a veil of tears enough for the species that inhabit it; denizens of the deep waters would do well to keep away from such a place, but perhaps whales are incurably reckless adventurers and D. H. Lawrence was right when he wrote (in 'Whales Weep Not!'): 'They say the sea is cold but the sea contains the hottest blood of all, and the wildest, the most urgent.'

Whales are not the only exotic marine creatures to have taken up my attention in the cold grey waters round the British coast. 'The time has come, the Walrus said, to talk of many things', and it was a young male walrus who hit the headlines in September 1981. Wally, as the press immediately christened him, inexplicably came to be wandering up and down the east coast of England far away from his rightful backyard in the shallow waters around the Arctic coasts. Walruses are not great seafarers, in the sense that they rarely move far from land. Occasionally they sail as far south as Iceland on icebergs, and there are about thirty pre-Wally trips to Great Britain by more adventurous individuals on record, the earliest reported by William Caxton in 1456 as being captured in the Thames! To me walruses are the most enchanting and mysterious of all pinnipeds, the family of flipper-footed animals that also includes seals and sea-lions. Gregarious, gentle souls whose

9

pups hold firmly onto their mother's necks as they move through the water, they are lovers of shellfish. We don't know the mechanism exactly, but somehow they suck the meat out of raw clams and other molluscs without swallowing the shells – and without benefit of hands or oyster knives! Hanne always says that I remind her of a walrus when I'm in a swimming pool (I take it as a compliment) and I must admit I love eating molluscs; heaven for me is a plate of *datiles*, the elegant brown mussels that the Spanish call 'sea dates', cooked in a garlic and onion sauce.

After great efforts by well-wishers who sought to help the obviously lost animal, Wally was caught and taken to Natureland at Skegness, a pleasant seaside marineland with long experience in handling stranded pinnipeds. Everyone – the animal protection societies, Natureland and Wally's host of instant supporters in Lincolnshire and farther afield – were concerned as to his future. He obviously couldn't stay in captivity. Walruses are not easy to keep, mainly because in concrete pools they grind away their tusks, exposing the root cavities and eventually developing serious dental abscesses. Tooth disease killed the majority of walruses that died in zoos. Also, suitable shellfish supplies are not easy to arrange in many places; in one day, a bull walrus may go through thirty to fifty kilos of molluscs, excluding the weight of their shells. Unfortunately Lewis Carroll's diet of bread, pepper and vinegar is relished only by walruses in the world through the Looking Glass! Hagenbeck's Zoo in Hamburg has been very successful in maintaining walruses by using a sort of substitute clam chowder diet of mashed mackerel, cream and oyster-shell grit and they have also thrived well in Holland at Harderwijk and at Sea World in San Diego. But no adequate facilities for Wally existed in Britain in 1981. He had been given cockles, mussels, whelks and sprats but had refused to dine. It was decided very sensibly to pack him off back to Greenland. The RSPCA organised everything and found Icelandair more than willing to give Wally a free ticket to the Arctic Circle.

10

Stefan Ormrod, Wild Life Officer of the RSPCA, phoned me to ask if I would go to Skegness to examine Wally shortly after his capture; there was some worry that he might have pneumonia because blood had been seen coming from a nostril. I travelled across country at once and arrived at daybreak on the Lincolnshire coast. I was in the marineland and standing by the pool which was Wally's temporary accommodation before any of the staff arrived. It was a wonderful moment for me – akin to the later experience of first handling a baby panda – to be alone with a young walrus who desperately needed a friend. Wally was covered in sleek, silver-gold hair and had a soft, broad muzzle sprouting rows of wiry ginger whiskers. One small tusk protruded from his mouth. The other, visible in photographs of him taken a couple of weeks earlier when he beached for a while lower down the coast, was gone – snapped off.

As soon as he saw me, Wally began 'talking' to me, making a haunting baying noise, rolling sad brown eyes and trying to climb up the wall to nuzzle me. As I walked round his enclosure he followed me closely, singing his forlorn song, and when I reached down to him he pressed hard against my hand with his sensitive muzzle. It was deeply moving. Hopping over the wall, I went up to him, crouched by his plump, barrel-like body and put my stethoscope to his chest, while this wild animal from the freezing seas of the far North behaved like a six-month-old labrador pup! Fortunately there was no sign of pneumonia – probably the bleeding, which had stopped, was related to the damaged tusk. I arranged with Katherine Parry, the local vet, for Wally to get a protective injection of oxytetracycline before he set off back home.

Wally returned triumphantly to the waters off Greenland, carried in a stout sea-lion crate and accompanied by RSPCA officials, and was released at a spot where other walruses were feeding. I guess he made up for lost time by diving straight down to the gravelly bottom and digging out the first Arctic clams that he'd eaten in weeks. As far as we know Wally is okay but. . . . When I was in Iceland shortly after his return, I was shown a clipping and a cartoon about the Wally affair taken from a local newspaper. In essence the point was that the Greenland esquimaux who hunted in the area where Wally was dropped off were tickled pink by the Englishmen's efforts in returning a live walrus to their neck of the woods. With any luck, they chortled, Wally will soon be tasty steaks and good leather hide if the spirits are with us. I hope the Gods of the esquimaux look compassionately on young Wally and send sudden gusts of wind to deflect the harpoons.

Some of the problems which I have faced as a doctor of marine and other wild animals are rather more fundamental and down-to-earth. Doctors of human beings have it easy when it comes to sex. Almost all the time they don't have any difficulty telling the males from females. Zoo vets aren't so lucky. I often pray that sex would literally rear its ugly – or really not so ugly – head for me. The problem lies in distinguishing males from females in a wide number of species ranging from birds such as flamingoes and parrots to young beavers and giant pandas. Of course the animal knows what it is and it can tell at the drop of a hat the difference between a cute little cocquette and a rather macho bloke. But how does the zoo vet do it?

We lack the animals' finely tuned senses of smell and, maybe, subtle comprehension of minute differences in behaviour and form, and of course we are not privy to the language of the beasts. Perhaps a lady parrot prattles on about the decline in the quality of modern sunflower seeds under the Tory government or about the latest fads in preening techniques, while the chauvinist male parrots swap rather risqué jokes about humans. ('Ever 'eard the one about the human that lived in a high-rise council flat, caught the number 37 to Putney every bleeding morning, six days a week, worked in the same office filing paper for twenty-five years, solid union man, same place in the Fulham ground every Saturday afternoon – thought he was *free*! Well, one day this bloody fantastic green-wing macaw gives 'im the old how's your father and says. . . .')

The secret life of animals is in so many ways closed to us, but knowing the sex of animals is obviously of great importance to anyone owning or working with them, let alone to the pair of vultures, say, who have spent ten infuriatingly infertile years in one another's company knowing that they most definitely did not turn one another on, all because some unwitting curator of birds thought they were a true and well-matched pair or, more frequently, because some bird dealer had sold them as a pair without having had a clue as to which, if it were so, was which. A pair of anything brings a far higher price than two males!

From time to time, therefore, sexing animals is an important part of our work. Young ostriches need to be examined manually by a hand introduced into the cloaca, beavers must be x-rayed, pandas need an anaesthetic for close inspection and the gender of certain lizards can only be sorted out by an abdominal operation. In recent years Andrew Greenwood has made a speciality out of sexing birds using the most direct and incontrovertible method – looking at the sex organs themselves by means of a fine fibre-optic laparoscope. This instrument, no thicker than a large-gauge hypodermic needle, is introduced under local or, in the case of obstreperous and mean-beaked parrots, general anaesthetic. Looking through the eyepiece on the laparoscope, one then comes face to face with either an ovary or a testis. It is a remarkably safe, quick and trouble-free technique and it has enabled us to establish breeding pairs with good hope of reproduction in zoos all over Europe and the Middle East.

When it comes to killer whales you would think that there wouldn't be much of a problem in the birds and bees department. The books say that there are distinct anatomical differences between the sexes. Males have triangular dorsal fins while females have backward-curving ones. But Cuddles, my first killer whale, had a backward-curving dorsal and he made it embarrassing plain, as he cruised around his pool upside down in what knowing old lady visitors to Flamingo Park would call 'an excited condition', that he was as butch as they came. The books also state that the external genitalia of males and females are different. Both have nipples, and the testicles of the male (as in dolphins, seals and sea-lions) are internal so there is no help in that direction, but whereas in the males there are two separate openings for the anus and prepuce, in the females the openings are closer together, both lying within a single deep trench in the skin. Sounds simple, doesn't it? Get your whale to roll over in the water or go paddling with him (or her) and count the slits. One equals female. Two equals male. Easy!

That was the state of the killer whale sexing game until 1980, when I was in Iceland doing checks on the six whales caught that season. Every December sees me on the bleak volcanic lava shore outside the little harbour town of Hafnarjordur, going over the new animals with a fine-tooth comb to make sure they are fit to travel to Japan, the USA or Europe and that they are insurable at Lloyd's. The whales are housed in a large pool close to the sea, and giving them medical examinations can be gruelling in ice-cold water with screaming winds and sleet-filled rain. Wet-suit gloves destroy my sense of touch. Working with bare hands is possible for only a few minutes before the cold bites excruciatingly through to the bone. The nervous new arrivals flail the water with their flukes and blind me with stinging spray or bruise my shins with a chop from a flipper. Jon Gunnarsson, the catcher, hands out snuff, which seems to repel the cold. Dan, my whale trainer assistant, built like the American footballer he once was, chatters his teeth behind blue lips as he struggles to hold a tail for my needle. The light is bad, the gloom of a sunless winter sky behind black storm clouds with nightfall coming by 3.30 pm at this time of year so close to the Arctic Circle.

When my precious sample bottles are full and safely labelled and on dry land, I must determine the sexes of the whales. Buyers of such valuable creatures know exactly what they want because exchanges later, even if possible with only four to six killer whales taken into captivity in the whole world each year, would be prohibitively expensive. Flying one whale between, say, Frankfurt and Tokyo costs at least $50,000. Sexing means bare hands plunged into the water and under the animals to feel for the all-important holes and slits. With bigger animals it means going down until my head is almost submerged. If the wind whips up a wave I go under for a second – oh God, why aren't I back in my home town of Rochdale spaying cats? I have to locate the orifices in question within ten seconds, otherwise my hands will seize up and stop functioning. Sexing a number of whales is a laborious affair with frequent breaks to blow on fingers, massage arms and hands, and take nips of brennevin, the ferocious Icelandic schnapps, from a hip flask.

In 1980 the sexing was carried out as usual and both Brynjolfur Sandholt, an Icelandic vet, and I were happy with our findings. There was no doubt about it: two males and four females. We checked and double-checked before they were allocated to their future homes in Canada, Spain and Japan. After some weeks of acclimatisation, when they were self-feeding strongly and with perfect blood counts, the animals were greased, carefully packed in foam and crushed ice and delivered by air to their distant marinelands.

All went swimmingly. I had just returned from Canada after accompanying two little whales, one male and one female, to Niagara Falls. It was New Year's Day 1981 and the telephone was ringing at 3 am in the morning, bringing me out of that first deep phase of sleep. 'Hurro,' said a voice, 'hurro, hurro.'

'Bugger off,' I replied irritably, convinced it was one of my friends preparing to wish me the compliments of the season and disguising his voice.

'Ha, please?' the voice continued uncertainly. 'Ha – Dr Tayrower?'

It wasn't a hoax I could hear a slight delay in the words and a hiss on the line. This was a very long distance and a genuine oriental.

'Yes, speaking,' I said, more compos mentis by now.

'Ah, Dr Tayrower. This is Magamushi, the marine*rand* in Japan. Togomoto speaking.'

Magamushi had bought two of the female whales from Iceland, I remembered. 'Oh yes, you have two new whales.' My heart missed a beat. Calls like this at odd hours shortly after delivery of animals usually meant trouble, sometimes a sudden death.

'Hai hai,' said the Japanese. 'We have two new wayuls.'

'They arrived OK?' I tried not to sound anxious. Dr Marty Dinnes had flown with those animals and hadn't reported anything amiss.

'Hai, yes. They allived OK, but we have plob*r*em.'

Well, at least they weren't dead, I thought. 'Please go ahead, Mr Togomoto.'

'Hai werr, you see, Doctor, we have elections here.'

Fully awake now and without being conscious of any effects from the sekt with which Hanne and I had seen out the old year, I struggled with that one. Magamushi is a municipal oceanarium. State money is involved. Politics? Politics are always intruding into animal affairs. Greenpeace had for the first time that year been very active lobbying, unreasonably in my view, against the taking of our killer whales, a species certainly not threatened with extinction. Perhaps that was it. 'You have elections,' I said. 'Er . . .'

'Ah yes. That is why I ling you, Dr Tayrower. Wrong elections. For sure we have a mayor.'

Maybe, I thought, that sekt was stronger than I imagined, but unless I was very much mistaken this fellow was giving me the results of his town council polls, which had apparently gone amiss in some way, and at a cost of around two thousand yen a minute in intercontinental telephone charges. If there is one thing I know and care nothing about it is local government politics in the land of the Rising Sun, and certainly not at 3 o'clock of a New Year's Day morning. 'I'm sorry, Mr Togomoto, but I'm in the dark.'

16

'Ha. In the duck?'

'I don't understand.'

The telephone line hummed to itself for some moments and then the Japanese spoke again. 'Ah Dr Tayrower, we have a mayor. We thought we had two *fe*mayors. We asked for two femayors.'

As if my caller's words were carefully phrased zen koans, I was instantly enlightened. 'Females, males,' I gasped. 'One of your females has turned out to be a male!'

'Hai, hai – yes. Without doubt we have seen an election of the wayul called Anna. Number one election, very wrong, very led when it froated on its back. Very wrong and led and . . .'

'Yes. Thank you, Mr Togomoto. I cannot understand it. Anna like all the whales was carefully checked.'

'Ah. Perhaps so, Doctor, but I have seen election, very wrong, very led . . .'

I was stunned as I put down the phone after agreeing to see whether a replacement could be arranged. How could there have been a mistake? What about the others – were there any other unexpected 'elections'? Within the next forty-eight hours I learned the worst: the Spanish whale, also thought to be a female, had suddenly and forcibly demonstrated its masculinity by popping several inches of phallus out of the 'vaginal' opening as it lay on its back, basking in the sunshine. The offending, inconvenient and impossible organ was photographed to prove it. There was no doubt about it: it was 'sayonara' to the accepted dogma on killer whale sexing.

In the 1981 season I decided to try again at manual sexing, if possible pushing my fingers far enough into the preputial orifice of 'males' to touch the tip of the penis. That would surely be a clincher. It would have been, but for the system of muscular pulleys that controls the S-shaped whale and dolphin penis. I did succeed in touching some penises in male killer whales in 1981 but discovered that sometimes the penis 'disappeared' on subsequent examinations, giving a distinctly female configuration. The whales could pull back or relax the position of the penis – a perfect mechanism for making fools of prying vets with chilly fingers!

The sexing errors of the previous year had caused much trouble and expense for all concerned and it was essential that I found a foolproof way of solving the problem. I decided to try tests which get right down to the basis of sexuality: chromosome examination. Males and females of all species have different chromosomes which can be recognised using special microscope techniques. Blood must be taken and white cells from it grown artificially in laboratory tissue cultures. When the white cells begin to multiply they are put on a glass slide, stained with dyes which pick out the details of the nucleus and examined under very high magnification.

To do all this requires, naturally enough, live white cells. My first attempts to get the tests done in the USA and Great Britain failed because, by the time the blood arrived at the lab, the cells had died. Iceland is a pretty isolated place. Then the laboratory of a hospital in Reykjavik came to our aid. They had all the requisite expertise and equipment for doing similar tests on humans with hereditary and congenital diseases and were willing to try their hand with whales. I supplied them with photographs of chromosomes from killer whales of known sex and they got to work. As a comparison I made the usual physical examinations. The Reykjavik hospital came up trumps in 1981, the whales' white cells grew well in the laboratory and behaved like proper little gentlefolk. Within four or five days of my blood sampling them we had definite answers and, as I suspected, they showed that once again we had not been correct with our manual probing in about twenty per cent of cases.

From now on as far as humans were concerned, the secret of the sex of a whale would lie in a tiny drop of blood. Dan was absolutely right when he said, as we watched the 1982 whales coming in 'Not having to stand so long sexing by hand in this damned water will stop us risking the sort of sex change that happens to brass monkeys!'

2 Panda Passion

'Mother Nature can put on a ruder show than a Soho sex shop,' said my companion. It was spring 1980 and I was in the Far East with Terry Nutkins. Terry, one of Gavin Maxwell's 'Ring of Bright Water' disciples in his youth and an experienced otter and marine mammal man, has been a close friend since we first met when the London Dolphinarium opened. The purpose of our journey to the Orient was to bring from Ocean Park, Hong Kong, to London a pretty Aduncus dolphin, the sort whose pale pink undersides become speckled with smudges of pigment as they grow older, thus earning them the name 'sea thrushes' among fishermen of the south China seas. After giving the animal a thorough medical and while waiting for the laboratory to complete its analysis of the dolphin's blood, we went by jetfoil down the China coast to the decaying Portuguese enclave of Macau.

It was the time of year for the migration of kingfishers, flashes of emerald-green flame over the dark water. The plum-pudding-shaped offshore islands with their rich encrustations of vegetation loomed in the low sea mist. Exploring the cobbled allies of the town with its smoke-stained, peeling stucco, scarlet Taoist temples, smell of spices, durian fruit, fish and night soil and sounds of distant ships' hooters and squeaking bicycle rickshaws, I was particularly interested in the traditional Chinese medicine shops. Gazing at their shelves full of bears' paws, deer antlers, rhino horns, dried and pickled animals and plants of a thousand varieties, I was reminded of the dragon's tooth that I had once pulled from a zebra's testicle in Singapore and the case of the sea cow's tears.*

*See *Doctor in the Zoo*.

The popularity in the Far East of what is essentially sympathetic magic for the treatment of human ailments and particularly sexual disorders is ageless. The grotesquely shaped mushrooms, plant tubers, marine invertebrates and bits of assorted mammal anatomy that are displayed in velvet-lined boxes or glass flasks sell for enormous prices. A kind of rare purple sea slug which, when dried, presents an appearance that would innocently outrage the sensibilities of Mrs Whitehouse, retails in China for around £200 sterling per drachm (one-eighth of an ounce). All these aphrodisiac panaceas, besides being expensive, have one other feature in common. Whether fungus, flesh of shellfish or horn of antelope, they resemble in some way, perhaps by stretching the imagination or indulging in a considerable degree of wishful thinking, the male or female (and occasionally both at the same time) human genitalia. Hence Terry's remark about Mother Nature's sex show.

There was a humid wind off the Pearl River estuary that scattered butterflies of black and phosphorescent blue as we continued our wanderings through the once wicked city that is now as down-at-heel and passé as an old whore. We came across first one and then several more of what we took to be Chinese pet shops – gloomy rooms with filthy cages lining the walls and standing in the doorways. The inmates of the cages weren't puppies, rabbits or hamsters but more exotic creatures. They were of only four kinds: leopard cats, eagles, fish owls and monkeys. Each pet shop seemed to deal in nothing but these. Of the usual Western pet shop accessories – dog leads, packets of ants' eggs, bird seed and the like – there was no sign.

Terry and I didn't like what we saw. The animals had eyes that were filled with desperation or were dull and fixed. Some of the leopard cats were plainly ill and emaciated. There was little evidence of food or water for any of them and no bedding. The living creatures on show certainly received none of the lavish care and elegance used in displaying the dead ones in the apothecaries' shops. Terry wanted to take some photographs of the squalid merchandise and made his intentions clear in gestures to the old, grey-pyjama'd Chinese shopkeeper who sat on a stool outside his shop. With a grin of gold and pyorrhoea he jumped to his feet and bowed us into the smelly interior.

Inside, a small and equally old lady sat impassively on an upturned box, surrounded by cages of silent animals. She was wearing a straw 'coolie' hat and black trouser suit and clutched a large basket as she watched us. As Terry adjusted his camera, the merchant pointed at his brown fish owl squatting in a perch-less, makeshift cage of chicken wire. Then he stared intently at me and, waving both hands in front of my eyes, made a karate-chop gesture in the air and jabbed a finger towards a back room which we could see through a partly opened door. The room was illuminated by another open door beyond, which gave onto a muddy courtyard. A young Chinese wearing an apron was bending over a wooden bench with his back towards us. The shopkeeper called to him and he looked up from his work, turning and giving us the sort of kow-towing obeisance never seen nowadays in Communist China or Taiwan. The old man repeated the sequence of pointing at the owl, me and the back room, along with the karate-chopping business. *'Bushi ming bai,'* I said. 'I don't understand.'

He picked up the cage by its wire handle, offered it briefly to me, then put it back on the floor and started karate-chopping for the third time. That finished, he came close to me, enveloping me in a mist of halitosis, and again looked intently at my face. The fingers came up and he pointed a fork of black-rimmed nails at my eyes. He was saying something in fast Cantonese – an unintelligible sales pitch, I assumed. Occasionally his eyes left mine and he looked at the fish owl, apparently making a reference to it of some kind.

'We don't want to buy your owls, squire!' Terry's loud voice echoed round the sad room. 'Tell the old bugger he'd get drummed out of Tib Street with a shambles like this.' (Tib

Street, the mecca for Manchester's pet owners, has its disreputable emporia but nothing to compare with this Macau version.)

The old man suddenly broke into a fleeting demonstration of his command of English. 'Fi honrad Hong Kong dollah,' he said, then reverted to Cantonese.

I shook my head vigorously. 'No, no. No want bird. *No queremos el buho.*' Perhaps a Macau Chinese with a bit of Portuguese might understand pidgin Spanish. The shopkeeper didn't flinch in his incomprehensible hard sell. He bent down and banged a fist on the owl cage and gesticulated yet again at my eyes and towards the back room.

All at once I saw what the young man was doing on his bench. He had half-turned and the sunlight from the courtyard fell on his moving hands. He was butchering. His bench was a block, dark with stains. A sharp hatchet of the sort used so deftly in place of a knife by Chinese butchers and sellers of fish was poised not over meat or fresh-caught grouper but above a small yellow and black heap of fur – a leopard cat, the handsome spotted feline known to the Chinese as 'Chin-ch'ien mao', or 'money cat', because its markings resemble old Manchu coins. The blade gleamed red as it cracked through the neck vertebrae and the head fell away. The man looked round, tilted his head in my direction with a broad, gum-baring smile and waved a gory hand.

Everything was now chillingly clear. This was no pet shop for Chinese who fancied something more challenging than a guinea-pig or a goldfish. Nor was it an oriental butcher's shop – Macau's answer to Dewhursts. This and the other similar establishments we had seen were just another kind of apothecary's, but instead of dispensing powdered mandrake, dried cuttlefish or wine containing eviscerated gecko, these pharmacists dealt in fresh medicines. Nothing could be fresher. The sympathetic magic approach to medicine holds that animals possessing appropriate natural abilities can yield valuable medicine for humans with certain ailments or weaknesses. That was why the old man had been going on about my eyes.

22

My vision is first-rate and unaided by spectacles or contact lenses, but he must have been suggesting that my sight would benefit from one of his prescriptions. Maybe he didn't like the look of something in my eyes or he was recommending a prophylactic against short-sightedness in approaching middle age. Whatever it was, the thing he reckoned would do the trick was eye, fresh from an animal possessing superb vision – the owl.

Should a customer come in complaining of rheumatism or lumbago he would reach then for the agile monkey and make a fresh infusion of its kidneys. The ferocious little leopard cats do wonders, he would say on the other hand, for those afflicted with nervousness or depression – a spoonful of brain three times a day before meals. Weakly children might benefit from being given daily morsels taken from the powerful eagle rather than, or sometimes as well as, cod liver oil and malt. And the young fellow in the back room would take the prescribed beast, kill it – I shudder to think how – and make up the potion on the spot. That was why the little old lady was waiting, just like my mother back in Rochdale after handing in her prescription for rheumatism pills at Mr Lane the chemist's shop. She would take a dose of whatever bit of the poor spotted cat she needed in a glass of water or wine right then and there.

Customers have to buy the whole animal even though they may only need some sinews, the brain or another organ. Despite the wide availability of more orthodox treatment methods, this ancient form of pharmacy still exists in many parts of the Far East, particularly among the Chinese communities, although it is banned in Hong Kong. It is still going great guns in Macau, however, as any visitor can plainly see.

Terry and I left the apothecary's shop feeling sickened and impotent. Anger seemed an inadequate response to an aspect of an ancient culture of which we knew nothing and had no part. 'How can that sort of primitive medicine do any possible good?' Terry muttered after we'd walked a long way in silence.

On the way I counted at least three restaurants specialising in wild animal dishes and particularly bear's paw soup. 'Anything works if you believe in it hard enough, I suppose,' I replied as we stood beneath the crumbling facade of the old colonial cathedral.

'Psycho-bloody-somatic!' The experience had doused Terry's abounding good humour. 'Roll on the revolution. The sooner Peking takes over here the better.'

He had a point – although many aspects of Chinese traditional medicine are being encouraged and expanded by the Communists, the use of animals in this way is dying out even in the rural areas of the People's Republic. 'To get over the culture shock,' I said, 'I suggest we should have a bottle of Tsing Tao at the Hotel Sintra and then get back to Hong Kong and our beautiful little dolphin.'

Soon after my return to England, echoes of the Macau visit came in a phone call from a well-respected businessman and confidant of the British Royal Family. Did I, he asked, know of any zoos or safari parks that might be 'culling' big cats or sea-lions? If so, there was big money to be made if I would kindly collect the sex organs and pop them in the deep freeze. He would collect them and send them off to the Far East for the traditional medicine market. 'They make up marvellous tonic wine called Szan Pien (three penises),' he explained. 'Organs of tiger, deer and sea-lion, together with the old ginseng. D'you think you can help?'

Three Penis wine is fairly easily obtained in Hong Kong, where I've often seen it on supermarket shelves. Whether or not it all really does contain what it claims I don't know, but I would hate to think I might contribute to making it as popular as Mateus Rosé and thus encourage one of the more bizarre corners of animal exploitation.

'No, I'm afraid not,' I told my distinguished caller. 'Why not try your local undertakers? They might be able to set you up with some really valuable spare parts. You could even try brewing your own and exporting it!'

He rang off.

24

Another spring, the sap rising, spring fever about. Birds and buffalos, country swains and crickets by the hearth – the thoughts of them all turn to romance. And even giant pandas, ascetic anchorites of the animal world, get the urge for a mere handful of days to live it up and go a-courting. In its native haunts, the misty forests of Szechuan, the panda prefers his own company for most of the year. He plods alone down tunnels he has bored through the dense tangle of mountain bamboo in a narrow band of altitude between 11,000 and 14,000 feet above sea level. Sunbirds fuss among the high foliage of birches and spruce and blood pheasants strut through the rhododendron and clumps of hemlock below.

It was in fact the spring of 1982 and, if our past experience was anything to go by, Shao-Shao, the female panda at the zoo in Madrid, would soon show what we considered to be signs of oestrus for two or three golden days. Her mate, Chang-Chang, who had been my first panda patient,* had shown not a scrap of interest in her amorous advances the year before. Always a benign and phlegmatic fellow who would allow me to listen to his chest and even stick a thermometer into his rectum while he relaxed after a lunch of Complan, eggs, rice and honey, he was, I was beginning to think, totally unimpressed by the opposite sex. Zoo panda males have frequently been like this. No wonder pandas are a small and endangered species. Was there perhaps a tendency for the males to be 'gay'? Or were they, perhaps, above base carnal desires – spending their secret days in the green and dripping gloom meditating on the deeper meaning of the philosophies of Confucius or Lao-Tse?

In February I had decided to try to kindle panda passion by playing chemical cupid. I had no wish to use hormones on Shao-Shao that might fundamentally affect her oestrus cycle but I saw no risk in giving shots of luteinising hormone to Chang-Chang. No mere aphrodisiac, this glandular extract stimulates the production of testosterone, the male hormone, by the testis. With no risk to side-effects I could perhaps make

*See Next Panda, Please.

the normally platonic Chang-Chang a bit more ardent. To be explicit, I was after, as Hanne suggested, a rather 'randy pandy'. Liliana, the veterinarian at Madrid, gave the series of hormone injections to Chang-Chang by trapping him as usual in the squeeze cage that encloses the weighing machine where his weight is daily recorded as a matter of routine. When the course was completed, Chang-Chang appeared as polite and proper as ever, but it would take the presence of a female panda in oestrus to prove whether or not he was now 'Jack the Lad', a young buck feeling his oats (or more, appropriately, his bamboo shoots).

Watching him in early March blandly scoffing his favourite imported British invalid food and then setting the empty bowl on his head as a helmet, sniffing my fingers diffidently when I had given him an apple or spending long hours napping in the fork of a tree, I could see precious little sign of ardour. Grub and naps – those were his principle interests. Sex, it seemed, had been sublimated; Chinese to the core, Chang-Chang was practising Buddhist self-denial and didn't give a damn for the pretty female who shared his grassy garden during the daytime. But she too was prim and proper: a more dangerous animal than Chang-Chang, at least for human beings, Shao-Shao didn't normally behave like a cuddly femme fatale. True, her interests embraced food and sleep, but they also included Jane Fonda-style aerobics in the paddock, climbing with the nimbleness of a Joe Brown and dedicated sunbathing.

I discussed the possibility of Shao-Shao coming into oestrus later in the month with David Jones, Chief Veterinary Officer of London Zoo. 'If it happens,' David said, 'we'll gladly anaesthetise our male and obtain a sample of semen by electro-ejaculation.' London's pandas had not proved compatible and their female had been afflicted with severe intestinal illness and a blocked fallopian tube that had, as in human ladies, to be 'blown clear' under anaesthetic. The London male had not got on at all well with the Washington female after being flown over to the USA for a much-publicised tryst. But he did have plenty of mature spermatozoa which, as far as scientists inspecting them under the microscope could tell, looked normal, vigorous and ready to go.

London's kind offer was too good to ignore. I 'phoned Dr Celma and Dr Cerdan, the directors of Madrid Zoo. If Shao-Shao came into oestrus and showed signs of sexual receptiveness, we would place an each-way bet. Chang-Chang, primed with his hormones, could do his stuff and Shao-Shao would also be inseminated, under anaesthetic, with semen from London. Now all we had to do was wait, and hope that deep inside the female panda's body an ovarian follicle or two were quickly ripening.

Mother's Day, 21 March, and things weren't looking too hopeful. In 1981 Shao-Shao had shown mild signs of what was possibly oestrus by this time. In Washington they had a week ago detected follicle maturation in their female, confirmed it by direct vision through a laparoscope under anaesthetic and inseminated her with semen flown in from London. After the ovulation they had witnessed a corpus luteum or yellow body forming where the egg follicle had been on the ovary. It wasn't possible to tell whether the yellow body was one of pregnancy or of non-pregnancy since they both look alike, but things seemed to be cycling properly and they knew for sure that they had injected the spermatozoa at the right time. It all augured well for a successful pregnancy in the American capital in autumn 1982. Were we in Madrid going to be left behind for at least another year? Was Shao-Shao still doomed to be a Chinese wallflower?

Then, on 25 March Antonio-Luis, Liliana's husband and the other resident vet at Madrid, phoned me in a state of high excitement. Something was afoot in the panda enclosure! Quite suddenly Shao-Shao had started to become much more vocally inclined. She was making loud mewing noises and she seemed more restless than usual. 'I think,' said Antonio-Luis, 'that this is the oestrus beginning.'

'Is the vulva enlarged?' I asked. We assumed that as with

27

many other species, female pandas would show swelling and congestion of the vaginal entrance during oestrus, but the private parts of these animals are difficult to see and few human beings had ever witnessed the physical alterations of a panda's heat period.

'I cannot see anything,' was Antonio-Luis' reply, 'but somehow I feel sure.'

The Spanish veterinarian had been closely involved with all aspects of the management of the pandas ever since they left China. I valued his opinion as a good observer and tireless worker. It might have been wishful thinking on his part but I thought it unlikely. 'When did you first hear her calling?' I asked.

'*Un poco* yesterday afternoon, but today it has continued all morning.'

It was worth a try. Shao-Shao just might be on the brink of ovulation. 'I'll contact London Zoo. Their veterinary officer and physiologist are standing by. As soon as London can get some semen, we'll be out on the next plane.'

John Knight and Harry Moore were up early at Regents Park on the morning of Saturday 27 March. John knocked out the male panda and then Harry inserted a specially built ejaculator electrode into the sleeping animal's rectum, pressed the button and in the twinkling of an eye collected some semen in a sterile test-tube. I was already on my way to Madrid. John and Harry came on the next flight, carrying the fresh sperm and also some that was deep-frozen having been taken at an earlier anaesthetising and deposited in London Zoo's panda sperm bank. The precious and hopefully life-giving liquid was transported in a cooled thermos flask protected by a special diluent and nitrogen gas. Essentially, the techniques employed in handling sperm samples from pandas are the same as for cattle, pigs and humans. Deep-freezing of bull semen and embryo transplantation in farm animals had been perfected many years before by Dr Steptoe (an old client of mine in Rochdale, who had the first Burmese cat I ever treated) engineered the birth of Louise Brown, the first test-tube baby.

By midday we had all assembled outside the panda enclosure. It was a perfect time for panda watching, with an eggshell-blue sky and air warm with the scent of rosemary. The prairie dogs were out for the first time that year, fussing round their burrows on the zoo lawns, and the oak trees of the Caso de Campo were blazing green with new leaves and noisy with woodpeckers, cuckoos and azure-winged magpies (the latter species remarkable in that outside Spain they are found only in eastern Asia). Our strategy had been discussed and agreed. First, we would let Nature take its course by mixing the two pandas together. Perhaps the still deadpan Chang-Chang would sniff pheromones on the morning breeze, perhaps the penny would drop in his mandarin's mind, perhaps. . . ! There was also of course the possibility that courtship might be scuttled by severe fighting, as had happened between the London male and the Washington female in 1980. After all, who are we to matchmake for animals? In the wild, panda males come from miles around when a female is in heat and there is much fighting and squabbling before she selects the one who takes her fancy. Whatever happened, it would be worth inseminating Shao-Shao afterwards in order to at least double our chances.

The panda keeper opened the two slide doors to the separate sleeping quarters. Blinking, the pandas shuffled out into the bright light. Chang-Chang was still wearing his food bowl as a helmet and looked ridiculous for one in the rôle of an amorous suitor. Typically, he made straight for his usual quiet napping corner, po-faced. Shao-Shao, also typically, was more active and did a few physical jerks on her lawn, rolling, stretching and somersaulting effortlessly. She mewed plaintively from time to time, something I had not heard her do so insistently before.

But an event much more remarkable was shortly going to occur, an event which has seldom been seen by human eyes. After ten minutes of fairly normal behaviour except for

Shao-Shao's vocalising, the female suddenly ambled up to her putative mate and stuck her bottom squarely and brazenly in his face. At that instant and to my utter astonishment and delight, Chang-Chang the continent, Chang-Chang the square, Chang-Chang the quintessential Chinese puzzle, came electrically to life. He jumped to his feet and quite plainly made a pass at the lady, trying to pin her down with both front paws. Shao-Shao slipped out of his grasp and then took up the same provocative position a few feet in front of him. Chang-Chang advanced again. Shao-Shao played hard to get and skipped away with a knowing gleam in her eye. Our hero was by now, however, a Lothario unleashed. He gave a mighty leap, brought the unprotesting female down, mounted – and forgot what it was all about!

I swear an embarrassed flush spread across the skin beneath his furry black and white mask. Like a coach turned into a pumpkin on the stroke of midnight, our bamboo-crunching Don Juan was suddenly a prim and prudish panda once again. Chang-Chang, the erstwhile rampant stud, now displayed a discomfited look. What on earth was he doing, I could almost see him thinking, in this ungainly position on top of another panda? How could it have happened? It was all rather embarrassing. Shamefacedly he climbed off and wandered over to his napping corner.

I and the other scientific voyeurs were delighted by progress so far. Even though, as I knew from my close-up view through binoculars, the critical consummation of this fickle affair had not occurred, the luteinising hormone was having an effect.

Shao-Shao wasn't going to allow her absent-minded suitor to give her such an ungallant brush-off. Mewing lustily, she loped over to the male, who was just settling down for what could not really be classified as a post-coital slumber, and presented her rear end once more. It worked as dramatically as before. All thoughts of sleep dispelled, Chang-Chang rose to his feet, Don Juan reborn, and grabbed the floozy. She flattened herself obligingly to the grass and he jumped on – and again, after a

30

few seconds seemed bewildered at the goings on and dismounted.

'Madre de Dios,' muttered Antonio-Luis. 'Necesita el libro
de instrucciones!' It certainly did look as if Chang-Chang
needed to brush up on the driving manual. Seven more times
during the next couple of hours the charade was repeated.
Seven more times Chang-Chang balked at the ultimate moment. Then, patience understandably exhausted, Shao-Shao
gave him a good cuffing round the ears and made it clear to us
that she wanted to go back to her indoor quarters.

The two pandas were put away and we prepared to take
matters into our own hands, literally. Tranquillised by a tiny
dart from a blow pipe, Shao-Shao was inseminated with the
sperm from London. Because we could not be certain exactly
when the egg or eggs would be released from the ovarian
follicle, the insemination was repeated on the next day,
Sunday, and again on the Monday, by which time Shao-Shao
had stopped her mewing. Chang-Chang was not totally
disgraced – he had at least shown willing, if not able, this year –
but he was no longer of any even passing interest to his mate.

Now we would have to wait and keep our fingers crossed that
one microscopic spermatozoon had made it, had against all the
odds got up into a fallopian tube, found an egg hanging
around (the timing was critical), penetrated it and begun that
most miraculous of all natural processes, the creation of a new
individual. Mouse, human or giant panda – the wonder of it
never ceases to astound me. We weren't absolutely sure how
long we would have to wait to learn whether the long-distance
mating had been successful. The gestation period in pandas is
not as well-known as it is in man and domestic animals.
Estimates ranged from 120 to 170 days and Mexico, who had
had a baby born after normal mating a couple of years earlier,
thought that 130 was probably the normal duration. But
no-one knew for sure.

It was decided to collect urine samples from Shao-Shao,
beginning on the day after her third and final insemination,

and send them in batches to the laboratories at Regents Park for analysis of hormone levels. Perhaps we would be able to detect pregnancy that way. It was a valuable opportunity to experiment anyway, though obviously nothing was known about the normal hormone output of wild animals which might have been compared with the results. Also, as I reminded Antonio-Luis, in 1981 the female panda at London had been declared pregnant after similar tests on her urine and much had been the interest and excitement of all concerned, particularly the media, who literally staked out the panda house in Regents Park ready for the big event certain to surpass even the famous 'Brumas' polar bear cub birth in newsworthiness. When the London panda eventually didn't produce any young, great had been the chagrin, particularly among the reporters and TV producers. Wisely, in 1982 Madrid agreed not to publicise any panda birth until and unless it actually happened.

The first weeks after the insemination were uneventful. Chang-Chang and Shao-Shao were their old selves – utterly platonic, somewhat distant acquaintances. The early urine samples showed nothing of note, and the hormone levels were of the same order as those in the few non-pregnant pandas in captivity which had been tested by London's method, but it was thought by the endocrinologists that positive cases wouldn't show up anyway before perhaps three months. April, May, June slipped by and then early in July we got news that we did not dare believe: London had found a distinct and significant hormone rise in recent samples from Shao-Shao. If she had been a human or a horse we would have rushed to prepare the labour ward or foaling stable, but was this test in giant pandas really reliable? Each day Liliana continued to collect a small bottle of urine from the drainage runnel in the floor of Shao-Shao's quarters. Whisked to London in His Hispanic Majesty's diplomatic bag, the samples continued to indicate that a tiny panda embryo was indeed making its presence known. It looked as though we really should prepare ourselves for the hoped-for great event.

The major facilities were already in existence in the zoo at Madrid. The panda house was well designed, constructed and equipped. Two senior keepers did nothing else but keep a round-the-clock watch on the two animals. There was a self-contained kitchen and entrance to the unit was across a disinfected foot-bath. It was a secure and peaceful place where a panda mother could surely give birth in quiet comfort. I discussed two further matters with Antonio-Luis and Dr Celma by telephone: the setting up of remote-control, closed-circuit television surveillance of Shao-Shao's den, and the standby preparations we should make in case any cub born was not accepted by the mother and needed artificial feeding.

The TV system was quickly organised and a sophisticated premature baby incubator was borrowed from a posh Madrid clinic to supplement the one permanently kept in the zoo veterinary hospital. More problematic was deciding what sort of baby milk to stock up with. The analyses of animal milks vary greatly from species to species. Sheep produce a liquid lower in fat and protein than that of cows but richer in sugar. Giving the wrong milk can have disastrous results – polar bear cubs accustomed to polar bear milk containing 31% fat and 10% protein fade away on the common or doorstep dairy pinta with 4% fat and 3.6% protein. Seals' milk contains very high amounts of fat but virtually no sugar, and any sugar-containing milk is usually lethal for their young. I have tables of milk analyses for a vast range of exotic species and by suitably augmenting cow's milk with extra cream, oil, protein powder, sugar or water I can knock up an acceptable substitute milk for anything from an Arabian gazelle to zebra.

But whereas I have on my books the requirements of even such an unlikely suckling as a blue whale calf (should you ever need the formula, it's 43.6% water, 56.4% total solids – 42% fat, 11.7% protein, 1.24% sugar), virtually nothing was known about the milk of giant pandas. I conferred with colleagues in

London and Washington, Peking and Madrid but there was no consensus of opinion, so it was decided to have various types of possibly suitable milk on hand, ready to switch quickly if signs of intolerance arose. From England I sent out SMA, Wysoy and Prosobee, soya-based baby milks ideal for infants who can't tolerate milk sugar. These I reckon were as good bets as any if Shao-Shao did produce a youngster and then wouldn't or couldn't rear it.

Towards the end of July I was in Salzburg in Austria to advise on an elephant of Circus Althoff which had a chronic swelling on its jawbone. With the elephant attended to, I spent a few hours looking round the old city and then went to the small zoo where they keep a curious freak eagle with a second pair of normal talons sprouting out of its breast. While in the zoo I received a phone call from Antonio-Luis, who had tracked me down after chasing me round Europe by telephone. 'David, *oyé*!' he said excitedly when I picked up the receiver. 'Incredible! I think Shao-Shao is going to have a baby very soon!'

It was the one hundred and fifteenth day after last insemination and Mexico City Zoo were predicting, if our tests were accurate, that we had only seven to ten days more to go. 'Why, what has happened?' I asked.

'I have caught a glimpse of the vulva and I think it is enlarging and relaxing. Also she is not behaving normally.'

'In what way?'

'She is not eating very enthusiastically, seems restless and she is moving straw from one place to another.'

Moving her straw! Making a bed prior to giving birth? That sounded more than just promising. I could not restrain a yell of delight. '*Fantastico, hombre*! But you are sure of the vulva?'

'I think so, David, but it's not easy to see, you know.'

'Keep in touch, *caballero*,' I said.

During the next few days, as we approached the magic date of 120 days post-insemination, I talked to Antonio-Luis every morning and evening to receive the latest reports. Ominously,

34

after the first sightings of a possibly pre-parturient vulva slackening off ready to permit, we hoped, the passage of a cub, the Spanish vet could detect nothing unusual at Shao-Shao's rear end. Had it been a false alarm? Oh Lord, please don't let false pregnancies be as common in giant pandas as they are in domestic dogs!

Certainly the female continued to act out of sorts and when the one hundred and twentieth day came and went without any sign of a delivery I began to have doubts, especially when Shao-Shao developed diarrhoea. A new dilemma arose: suppose she was ill? Poor appetite, restless, abnormal behaviour, diarrhoea, and in an animal whose mate had a long history of gastro-intestinal upsets: I must beware of putting everything down to a possibly illusory pregnancy and missing the onset of disease. Imagine sitting back, waiting for a baby and doing nothing, and then finding we had lost the mother from untreated illness! But what dare I do to a possibly pregnant panda? Things didn't look grave enough yet to risk complications with any foetus through use of an anaesthetic. Many, many drugs are taboo or at least better not administered during pregnancy in animals as well as humans. I decided to take a prudent, conservative path. 'Give Shao-Shao a course of ampicillin in her food,' I instructed. This modern drug would tackle any bugs that might be troubling her insides without producing side-effects.

Shao-Shao's motions improved after the ampicillin and she seemed to return more or less to her usual demeanour although her appetite remained rather fickle. The 130-day point was reached and passed and then 140. Still nothing. And no more glimpses of an enlarged vulva. By 150 days my doubts were firmly entrenched. We were three weeks overdue by Mexican calculations.

Of course, for all we know, the phenomenon of delayed implantation of an embryo might occur in giant pandas. This natural mechanism, whereby after fertilisation an egg hangs around for a variable period before implanting in the uterus and getting started on pregnancy proper with progressive development of the foetus, occurs in such species as bears, badgers, otters, armadillos and certain deer. It results in a gestation period of flexible length and is useful to animals which may need to wait for optimum climatic and other environmental conditions before bringing forth their offspring. Perhaps the reports of pandas going up to 170 days were true. I hoped so but didn't really believe it.

With everything humdrum and boringly normal in the panda house by the end of August, I could delay a scheduled trip to the Middle East no longer. Chris Furley, our assistant, who is based permanently at the zoo at Al Ain, was just recovering from a bad attack of virus hepatitis. He needed a vacation to recuperate and I had to stand in for him at the zoo in the United Arab Emirates. Soon I was immersed in the welter of day-to-day problems in the large collection of exotic animals kept in the oasis on the Oman border, in the gardens of the innumerable sheiks' villas as well as in the vast zoological park. From 6 am to 6 pm every day there was a continual stream of patients to attend to. Bedouins coming in from the desert with hunting falcon ailments, gibbons, giraffes, ante-lopes, tigers, gorillas and ostriches suffering from problems peculiar to a hot and arid environment and of course the inevitable queue of Afghan, Pathan, Baluchi, Irani and Sudani keepers with headaches, sore eyes, stomach pains and cut fingers for my ministrations.

By a stroke of luck I was in the office of the director, Mr Bulart, at 10 am Emirates time on 4 September when the telephone rang. It was Hanne calling with great news: panda twins had been born at Madrid during the night. It was the one hundred and sixty-second day and I was four thousand miles away. I couldn't leave the Middle East for another eleven days at least; I didn't know whether to laugh or cry.

Luckily Andrew was in Europe and even as I spoke to Hanne was waiting at Ringway Airport in Manchester for the shuttle down to Heathrow to catch the next Iberia flight to Madrid. I immediately 'phoned him in Ringway's executive lounge and caught him just before he boarded the aircraft. We discussed all possible aspects of management of the pandas during the critical post-natal period. It was difficult to concentrate on the falcons with bumblefoot and snuffly noses that morning.

Newborn baby pandas are pink little grubs, not in any way resembling the furry, black and white 'bear' cubs one might imagine. Proportionately to other mammals, they are far smaller than their parents, and in this they resemble true bears such as the polar. They have a sparse covering of uniformly pale-coloured hair and long tails. The Madrid twins were typical of their sort; one weighed about ninety grams and the other just over a hundred grams. From the start it was obvious that the smaller one was not very acceptable to Shao-Shao. She concentrated her attentions on the other and it was decided to remove the ninety-gram cub to attempt artificial rearing in the incubators. Despite a major effort by the assembled Spanish and English veterinarians, the little panda died at two days of age. Andrew brought samples of its organs back to England, where pathology tests showed that the cause of death had been an acute pneumonia caused by a bacterium, the sort of malign germ that sometimes causes epidemics of disease in human hospitals and leads to children's wards being temporarily closed.

Despite this setback there was much to be satisfied with concerning the other cub. Shao-Shao tended and nurtured it with great affection. She seemed to have abundant milk in her breasts and the infant rapidly put on weight. The maternal experience mellowed Shao-Shao's temperament and she became much more amenable and gentle towards her keepers and veterinarians. By the time I returned from Arabia and had the chance to get to Madrid, things looked very promising for a natural, uneventful rearing of the young panda. After two months it looked like a proper mini-panda should look, with a rich black and white coat and dark eyes that had only just opened. Its tummy was plump and it scratched, rolled and wriggled contentedly as it lay on its mother's warm belly. The TV monitor recorded its every action in thrilling coloured detail but nothing was more breathtaking than quietly opening the thick wooden door of Shao-Shao's den and peeking in directly at the still only small (perhaps 1,500-gram) panda. *Viva el oso panda de Madrid!*

3 Monkey Puzzles

The zoo vet hasn't always got the luxury of an operating theatre and well-equipped veterinary hospital like that at Madrid when it comes to emergencies, and often I feel like a battlefield medic having to make do and mend under fire. It's a great tribute to the fitness and natural powers of healing of wild animals that so many operations carried out in the far from ideal place with bad lighting, little or no assistance and sometimes improvised equipment do go remarkably well. Large animals such as elephants, giraffes and camels are still generally best dealt with in situ in their stables, paddocks or fields. It would rarely be possible, even if desirable, to hospitalise such a patient. But smaller creatures can usually be tranquillised in their quarters and then removed to a hospital area – if it exists. Even the smallest beasts, though, sometimes require on-the-spot surgery.

Chessington Zoo has changed immensely under its new management, with an excellent examination room and post mortem laboratory among other things having been built in recent years. Despite its image within the zoological establishment as a 'commercial' funfair-cum-small-zoo that cannot be taken seriously, Chessington has a first-class breeding record in a wide range of exotic species from sea-lions to otters to lemurs to beavers and a dedicated staff of young keepers, many of whom are as good as any you will find in European or American zoos. Its percentage incidence of disease is lower than Regents Park and it is steadily replacing old and out-moded exhibitions with effective new ones, using money it earns and not from government handouts. In the days before Chessington possessed a special veterinary clinic with hydraulic operating table and the like, I had to tackle operations in the same way that I had done at Belle Vue Zoo in Manchester twenty-odd years before, but without benefit of a fully-equipped surgery fifteen miles away as had been the case when I lived in Rochdale.

At Chessington in pre-clinic days animals had to be operated on in their own houses or else in some ersatz theatre in a food kitchen or barn or curator's office, frequently with no time to clean, disinfect and warm up the surroundings. One can argue that there were advantages in those good old days, which ended with the advent of the NHS, when the family doctor would remove an appendix on the scrubbed kitchen table, but they were outweighed by all the considerable disadvantages. With zoo veterinary work on small species the same is true, but when there is no alternative I do confess to secretly revelling in the need to fall back on the old fundamental principles of successful surgery: speed, efficient anaesthesia and a good technique. These are infinitely more valuable than gadgets and gear, shadowless operating lights, electro-cauteries, masks and gloves and a bevy of beautiful RANA nurses mopping one's brow. And a fast operation is more important than worrying about dust in the air or the lack of sterile drapes to surround the operating site; soap and water and skin disinfectant will suffice where time is of the essence. Post-operative infections are very rare in my experience and when they do occur are a nuisance rather than a serious threat to life.

Caesar, the male Capuchin monkey at Chessington, had a mate called Cleopatra, and when she became pregnant Chris, the head primate keeper, didn't expect any trouble. Monkeys usually give birth without difficulty and I find that I am only called about twice a year to give obstetric assistance to primates and need to do a Caesarean section perhaps once every two years in apes or monkeys. Monkey mums-to-be keep fit and do their exercises! When her six-month gestation period approached its conclusion, Chris watched carefully for the first signs of labour in Cleopatra. An experienced primate man, he knew what to watch for: a discharge of waters, contractions and the speedy presentation of a baby looking at first like a drowned rat. It would be a brief, undramatic affair. More likely than not, it would happen at night or during the day just when he nipped to the loo. On his return Cleo would be proudly grooming the new infant, its umbilical cord chewed off by her and hanging down, a couple of inches of glistening pink cord. She might well have started scoffing the lump of placenta that quickly followed the baby.

But it didn't happen that way. Chris spotted Cleo's first contractions early one morning. She was definitely bearing down, but there was no sign of placental water loss. He waited an hour and, when there was no change, telephoned me.

'No sign of any discharge at all?' I asked.

'None,' came the reply.

'OK leave her another couple of hours but ring me before if there is any sign of blood without the baby making its appearance.'

Exactly two hours later Chris 'phoned again. 'No change,' he reported. 'Contractions regular every six to seven minutes. Still no signs of water or blood and she's behaving otherwise as if she hadn't a care in the world.'

I decided to wait. It is a mistake to interfere too early in the birth process of animals. 99.9 per cent of creatures, particularly wild ones, deliver their young unaided by the prying fingers, instruments or drugs of well-meaning humans. Doing nothing can often be the wisest and safest form of treatment. Precipitate action can cause innumerable problems. The trick is spotting the one-in-a-thousand case that needs early intervention if mother and baby are to be safe. Chris's accurate observation and my knowledge of monkeys gave me confidence in acting Brer Rabbit for a while longer.

Half a day passed and Cleo progressed not one whit but then she didn't decline either. By the evening I had to make another decision: to let things take their own course through the night, ask Chris to sit up with the little monkey or bring matters to a head by forcing labour to a speedy conclusion. It isn't easy 'guesstimating' Nature's intentions and while a dead baby is awful enough, a dead mother is heartbreaking. Nevertheless, enlightened zoo management requires that animals are treated as individuals, not as machines. A uterine cervix that relaxes in its own good time is usually to be preferred to one that is forcibly expanded. A natural birth that 'paces' itself gives the body time to adjust and minimises trauma. With Cleo showing no sign of pain, discomfort, illness or discharge, I told Chris to go home and phone me as soon as he came to the zoo next morning. The phone rang at 7.30 am. 'She's much the same as yesterday. No discharge but the contractions are very weak and widely spaced.' The primate keeper sounded upset. 'She's been at it a day now.'

There are no fixed rules in such matters but twenty-four hours in the second stage of labour is the limit as far as I am concerned in monkeys. Now I had to interfere. I breakfasted on Marmite toast sandwiches while I drove through the rush-hour traffic in Chobham and Byfleet on the twenty-mile journey to Chessington from the house near Bagshot which has been my home and the practice's southern office since I moved down from Lancashire. As is my custom, I used the travelling time to go over mentally the possibilities of what might lie ahead: courses of action, snags, how, where, which and so forth. Past difficulties with monkeys in labour. Special points concerning Capuchins. Anatomy? Physiology? Anaesthetic? A mental check-list of instruments needed. What drugs were in the zoo dispensary? What was I carrying in the Bag? By the time I turned into the zoo gates I was fully rehearsed in my head. The real thing would be just a familiar re-run.

Cleo sat calmly in a corner of the Capuchin house, hands folded across her swollen stomach. Her fur was glossy black except for a silver-white tonsure crowning the face that wore, like all Capuchins, a perpetually surprised expression. She raised her eyes and grimaced toothily at me as I watched the feeble contractions within her abdomen. She didn't push at all.

The muscles of the uterus were tiring of their efforts to expel the reluctant baby. Whatever I did, she needed anaesthetising straight away. Chris caught her easily in a sort of heavy-duty butterfly net and then, taking both her arms firmly behind her back, held her securely in a full nelson while I injected half a cc of ketamine solution into her thigh. Within a couple of minutes she was unconscious and I disinfected my hands in order to perform an internal examination. As I suspected, the cervix was hardly open at all. With the tip of my little finger I could feel the intact placental 'bag of waters' pushing into it from the far side. Placing my stethoscope to Cleo's chest and stomach, I quickly located two distinct heart sounds. Mother's fast. Baby's even faster, but completely normal. Only one thing for it: a Caesarean. I would do it at once in the old quarantine room.

A little while later, Cleo was lying on a piece of plastic sheet covering a wooden food-preparation table. A keeper stood at my side holding the stainless steel bowl that contained a few basic instruments, scalpel, forceps, scissors, needles and sutures under the light from one fluorescent strip in the ceiling.

After topping up the injected anaesthetic with a further dose, I tied Cleo flat on her back with four pieces of string fixed between her limbs and the table legs. Then I washed her belly with water and povidone antiseptic. For scrubbing up I used the quarantine kitchen sink and, lacking sterile towels, prepared to operate with wet hands, shirt sleeves rolled well up. One stroke of the scalpel divided skin, muscles and silvery peritoneum. The pale blue mass of the womb rose into my incision. I chose a spot over the head of the foetus within and carefully cut the uterine wall. Taking a hold of the tiny skull between finger and thumb, I hauled the baby out and then peeled the placenta from its attachment. The womb began to shrink down at once while I massaged the infant with my hands and wiped mucus from its nose and mouth. It responded by writhing and screwing up its face. I tied off the umbilical cord, cut it and handed the baby to Chris. A round needle and a

43

length of fine catgut were needed next. I inverted the edges of the uterine incision and put in a watertight continuous line of stitching. There hadn't been more than a saltspoonful of bleeding. I closed the muscles with more catgut. It is important to pick up the peritoneum while doing this and the last stiches are fiddly to insert – thank God for a small hand when operating on such minute creatures! Finally I placed a line of individual dacron sutures in the skin. It was all over in twelve minutes.

As Cleo began to rouse from the effects of the ketamine, the baby lay in a shoebox under an infra red lamp, squeaking lustily. It later transpired that Cleo hadn't enough milk to raise the baby who was christened, appropriately enough, Mark Antony. So the keeper reared him on Ostermilk and baby-food and eventually re-introduced him to his parents and the rest of the Capuchin colony. He is still at the zoo in Chessington, a fine specimen of his kind and none the worse for his delayed and unpromising arrival into the world.

It wasn't a difficult or unique operation and Capuchins aren't a rare species with the superstar charisma of pandas or birds of paradise, but when I see him on my weekly inspection visits pulling faces at the crowd or leaping fluidly from branch to branch with a bunch of mealworm titbits clutched in one hand, I get the feeling of secret exaltation that is the real, unsurpassable reward in being GP to wild animals.

Some exotic animals – gerbils, hamsters, budgerigars for example – make very good pets. But the majority are not suitable for keeping by private owners on the whole and in Britain the Dangerous Wild Animals Act and conservation legislation have mercifully reduced the number of people who keep lions in their gardens or crocodiles in their bathrooms to a mere handful. It isn't the same overseas, where the rich, flamboyant or eccentric can still indulge their fancies for rare creatures; I recently looked at a young lion given as a gift to the King of Spain by a well-known singer, who may think he knows a thing or two about singing but can't have employed much grey matter when picking a prezzy for HM Juan Carlos. Where did he imagine the King could keep such a creature? Of course, it ended up in the zoo in Madrid where it sits in a quarantine cage while everyone (except the singer) worries over its future. How to graft it into an already established and harmonious social group? Should it, be kept alone to avoid the inevitable and sometimes fatal fighting? Not a happy thought. But folk like showbiz personalities with their grand gestures and eyes on the publicity machine don't need to worry about such things. Only the lion, the zoo director and the vet are left to sort things out after the press photographers and PR mouthpieces down the last glass of champagne, gobble the last free canapé and go.

It's even worse in the Middle East. At Al Ain, unwanted, totally unexpected gifts of animals which have been received by sheiks are passed on to the zoo, usually without warning, almost every week. Tiger cubs, leopards, ostriches, monkeys, birds of prey – given by the ignorant rich to the ignorant rich – end up in makeshift accommodation behind the scenes. We never euthanase such living presents: just swear, grit our teeth and start looking for somewhere to park the bewildered creatures.

Primates are most definitely not to be recommended as private pets, although there are rare exceptions. One such is another Capuchin monkey, 'Cappy', who lives in Manchester. I first met the little fellow in 1974 when he was about two and a half years old and had just been purchased by the Bunting family. He at once became, and still remains, as well cared for and integrated a member of the family as any of the humans – or the dog. Nothing but the best for Cappy: he demanded and got everything a Capuchin who thinks he's a human might demand, and his quarters in the kitchen were a focal point of the Bunting's daily life. Cappy Bunting was very much master in his own house and he patently revelled in it.

About a year after his arrival, Mrs Bunting telephoned me to say she was worried about the little Capuchin. On the frequent occasions that he was out of his cage and roaming free, instead of as normal sitting beside the fire, watching television or grooming the dog, Cappy had taken to spending a long time in the scullery, drinking from the cold water tap. He was also vomiting frequently and losing weight. I went out to examine him. Already Cappy was quite clear as to who was one of the family and who wasn't. Vets definitely were not, and I was scolded severely as he sat on his mistress' lap while I listened to his chest and poked fingers into his abdomen. He tugged at my ophthalmoscope while I peered into his eyes which, thank goodness, were clear and healthy right through from front to back, for I had a growing suspicion as to the cause of Cappy's ailment. Taking a paper test strip, I touched it against the end of his penis. The paper at once turned blue, indicating the presence of sugar. Cappy, as I had guessed, was a diabetic.

Diabetes is not uncommon in wild animals and I have had cases in camels, kangaroos, various sorts of cats and bears. Many cases in captive animals, I believe, are due to a dietary fault, particularly where they are being hand-reared on artificial milk. It may be too much or the wrong sort of sugar in the milk or in some cases excessive protein. Whatever the exact cause, it can produce disastrous effects including irreversible cataracts in the lenses of the eyes. In early life Cappy had suffered a bone weakness and had been persuaded to accept the appropriate medicine each day for many weeks by mixing sugar with it. I wonder sometimes if too much of this sweetener was the cause of his later diabetes.

So how to tackle a monkey with diabetes? Particularly a monkey who adored sweet things, who consumed great quantities of grapes, sultanas and peaches and for whom Mrs Bunting baked little cakes, saved the finest first cut of golden-brown skin of the family's baked rice pudding and bought a quarter of a pound of jelly babies or some Toblerone as a Saturday treat? Insulin injections work as effectively in animals as in man but it wasn't likely that Cappy would take very kindly to once-daily pricks with a needle. At two and a half years old he already possessed a muscular body and dangerous teeth, and he ruled the roost in the kitchen. No-one was disposed to argue if he decided he didn't like something. Quite a martinet, Cappy was nevertheless deeply loved by everyone else in the family, except perhaps the long-suffering dog; they were deeply alarmed by my diagnosis but equally utterly determined to do everything necessary to combat the diabetes.

Many owners of animals simply haven't got the will power to put their pets on to strictly prescribed diets. They 'forget' the chocolate drops that an obese pooch with heart disease and on half a tin of reducing diet and a raw carrot per day is slipped every evening before going to bed. They cannot see any harm in the parrot with diarrhoea and the bland diet of yogurt and pobs (which it obviously hates, the way he's giving them filthy looks) being given a secret sliver of tangerine in order to get into his good books. We don't have any trouble of this sort among the professionals in zoos, I might add. The Bunting family surprisingly proved also to be very professional in rigorously applying the diet I at once outlined for Cappy. No sweet fruits, no chocolates or sweetmeats, no sugar. Cappy would have to eat meat, tinned dog food, egg, cheese and vegetables. The only fruit I would permit was a little tomato. I don't think the Buntings ever 'cheated' once.

There are anti-diabetic drugs such as tolbutamide which are taken by mouth instead of injection and work well in many human diabetics but they don't generally reduce the blood sugar of other diabetic species. An exception, as one might imagine, are the non-human primates. I decided to try Cappy on tolbutamide. I needed to arrive at a dose which in conjunction with the low-sugar diet was just enough to keep Cappy's urine free of sugar. I supplied Mrs Bunting with a bottle of test strips and got her to dip one into a puddle of Cappy's urine twice a day. She was to adjust the tolbutamide tablet dosage until there was no blue colour produced. Within a week Mrs Bunting had found the optimum dose of the drug and I arranged for her to continue thereafter doing weekly checks in case, as was likely, the monkey's requirement of tolbutamide altered.

The change in Cappy after beginning the treatment was dramatic. His thirst and vomiting vanished and he began to put on weight. His family faithfully kept up the urine screening, drug dosage and careful diet and he grew into an otherwise normal, powerful, adult male Capuchin. Now, nine years on, he's still going strong and free of any apparent side-effects from the diabetes. Mrs Bunting probably knows more about nursing a diabetic monkey than anyone else in England and Cappy certainly knows he's head of the house in the best of homes.

It was in Manchester a few years before Cappy came on the scene that I met another exotic pet kept in quite different surroundings. It was the property of a Professor of Medicine at Manchester University Medical School. Why he kept the beast I shall never know, for one day the Professor had a heart attack and died and the police called me to go as soon as I could and do something about a 'bloody great ape' that was locked in an upstairs room of the deceased's house and terrorising the undertakers who were laying out the body. Apparently it was beating on the walls and bringing down the plaster.

The Professor had lived alone in Fallowfield, and the Victorian house of smoke-black and stone with ledges and windowsills frilled white with pigeon droppings was gloomy inside, full of dusty bookcases and worn velvet chairs. It smelled of damp, Vick lozenges and pipe tobacco, and in a glass jar on a table in the hall was the pickled breast of a negress erupting with a grotesque carcinoma. The faded sepia of its label said 'Gabon 7/1/19'.

The undertaker's assistant met me in the hall and took me up. I could hear the racket even as I began to climb the stairs. There was a riot, a mutiny in full swing, a bear-garden somewhere up there. The howling, banging and crashing of objects was incessant. On the landing, which was lit by a dim bulb in a be-cobwebbed red glass lampshade, I looked at the door behind which pandemonium reigned. In the threshhold of a nearby doorway stood the undertaker in his working overall, smelling of formaldehyde and looking as if he had seen a ghost. 'It's going to break out, I'm sure,' he said, waving a pair of rusty tweezers at me. 'You'd better do something quick, friend, or it'll be out and no mistake.'

'Has he – the dead man – no relatives?' I asked. The 'thing' was beating on the door now and dust was puffing in little spurts from around the frame.

'None. All alone he was, the Prof. Except for that thing.'

'Any idea what it is?'

'Bloody great gorilla, I believe.'

I frowned as the hairs on the back of my neck sprang to attention; 'it' certainly made as much noise as a big silver-back, but I was going to have to open the door to get a shot at it with the dart gun. 'You get on with your work,' I said to the funeral pair. 'I'll be OK taking things quietly on my own.'

The undertaker and his assistant retreated, closing their door and leaving me feeling like a character in *The Murders in the Rue Morgue*. The door behind which 'it' lay, or rather sounded distinctly to be laying into things, had no key in the lock. I crouched down to look through the keyhole. I could see nothing but a patch of peeling wallpaper on a far wall. Gingerly I turned the door knob and pushed a little – definitely locked. I had to assume that 'the thing' could not have bolted itself in. The key must be somewhere on this side. It was nowhere to be found on the landing. I tapped on the other door. 'Any sign of a key in there?' I shouted over the din.

'No, not here,' come the faint reply, almost drowned by what now sounded like 'it' beating a billet of wood against the floorboards and, what was more, precisely to the stately beat of the Dead March from *Saul*. Or so I imagined.

From the kind of noise its feet made on the floorboards and the vocal sounds, I was fairly certain it wasn't anything as big as a gorilla, but it could have been a chimp or maybe a baboon –

both very dangerous animals if roused. A chimp is as strong as six grown men and has a bite as bad as a mastiff's. A baboon can take on a lion and has been known to keep advancing even against shotgun fire. Oh dear, I thought as I went downstairs and back to the car to fetch the Bag and something to open the door with, no wonder there isn't a copper around. If it had been a hoodlum or a maniac with a knife holed up in the house the place would have been stiff with constabulary. As it was, Sergeant Bumble had passed the buck to me and now I was on my own, feeling like Oliver Twist in a house with a corpse, Mr Sowerberry and Noah Claypole – and King Kong on the side for good measure!

My car boot contained several handy objects including the stainless steel chisels and a mallet with which years earlier I had removed the great tooth from Mary the elephant at Belle Vue.* They should make mincemeat of breaking a lock. In fact, looking at the collection of extraordinary veterinary gear – stainless steel wire with handles that could whistle through dense bone and amputate a leg in seconds, a balling gun for delivering giant pills down large animals' throats that looked like a baseball bat with a metal-filled end, and a collection of evil-looking knives, files and pincers for trimming overgrown hooves – one could forgive an inquisitive policeman should he ever stop me at dead of night on the way back from an emergency (with blood on my clothing, undoubtedly) for gazing with considerable interest at this little lot: ' 'Allo, 'allo, 'allo. What 'ave we 'ere? Garrottes, clubs, instruments of mayhem and burglarious tools?' 'Well, officer, not exactly. These, for instance, are for taking teeth out of elephants.' 'Ho, ho, ho, ho – then do you mind blowing into this bag, sir?'

I loaded a syringe with the fastest-acting paralytic drug I had – suxamethonium – a big dose just in case of a surprise. Professors of Medicine who'd been to Gabon before the war just might have brought back a missing link! Walking back to the house, I looked up at the window which must have

*See *Zoovet*.

belonged to the room in question. It was completely covered on the inside of the glass with rusty iron mesh. Back on the landing, the door to the room where the corpse lay opened a crack and two pairs of eyes stared out. 'Have you done it yet?'

'Not yet. Get back in. I've been to get my stuff.'

The door was hurriedly closed. I do not have illusions about myself in a Starsky and Hutch rôle, nor do I fantasise (even as I begin to go bald) of having anything of Kojak in me, but it did seem to me that the approved American detective way of kicking in the door and dropping to a crouch, legs apart and gun held in both hands, was at least worth trying first. It had the element of surprise which would be lacking if I started chiselling. As 'it' came charging out I would let it have the flying dart straight in the chest or belly (I had selected a short needle which wouldn't do much physical injury but with a barb to ensure that it held on).

I treble-checked the dart gun, made sure the safety catch was off – no more cock-ups like the puma/Great Dane fiasco of which I have written before* – and practised the movements in slow motion a few times. I was now ready for an SAS-style entry. I positioned the gun dead centre and held the trigger lightly. Okay, you guys! So far so good. The sweat dripped off my brow and it wasn't because it was hot. I didn't feel very SAS – more like the Royal Army Veterinary Corps, but then they don't go round kicking doors in. I breathed in, lifted my right foot and smashed it forward so that the heel of my shoe hit the door just below the knob. The door shuddered, the knob dropped of, but the door did not fly open. I repeated the attack – nothing doing.

So much for Starsky and Hutch. The heavy wooden door possessed a very solid lock. The noise in the room was continuing unabated. Irritated, I picked up the door knob, fiddled with it and eventually managed to fit it back on to its spindle. Right, it had to be chisels. I jammed my longest chisel into the gap between door and frame close to the lock and

*See *Going Wild*.

began hitting it as hard as I could with the mallet. The creature on the other side joined in. Between blows I could feel it pounding back at me. Well, with two of us working at it this should be a doddle! With a splintering crack the lock suddenly gave, and I heard it crash to the floor inside. There was a metallic scraping noise as 'it' picked it up and then a thud as I visualised the creature hurling it against a wall. The door, mercifully still held by the catch below, should now be free. I tested, heart thumping, by turning the knob and pushing just a millimetre. It was open.

I pulled it tight shut and hung on to the knob like grim death while I re-ran through my memory all the old Elliot Ness and FBI films I had watched, rather in the way that a drowning man is said to see his whole life flash before him in an instant. How did it go? Open door by means of knob, fling it wide with left hand and flatten myself against landing wall with gun in right hand. Peep round door and let 'it' have it.

I squeezed the gun-butt tightly, turned the door knob and shoved it inwards with all my might. The door flew back as I pressed myself against the wall. At once a brown mass of fur came shooting out onto the landing. Screaming diabolically, the mass sprouted arms and legs and leapt up onto the banisters at the head of the stair-well. I swung the gun round and pointed it at the creature.

Before me squatted a travesty of a pig-tailed macaque monkey. One eye bulged blind and orange-coloured from its socket, the mouth snarling agape showed long, brown, deformed teeth, the belly was swollen and hairless and the toenails were so overgrown that they were curling into corkscrews. Despite all this it was still an immensely strong-looking animal – almost a cube of muscle as it crouched, glaring at me with a mixture of fear and hatred. I moved to one side to avoid a ricochet if the syringe bounced back, breaking the barb at such close range, and squeezed the trigger. At the same instant the monkey gave a great scream and hurled itself at the door behind which the undertakers were at work.

Wrenching the knob, it burst inside. My syringe buried itself in the landing wall, showering plaster down the staircase. Now the howls were human ones. Out of the room of death the undertaker and his assistant came hurtling as if pursued by the Grim Reaper himself. 'Good God, it's after us!' yelled the undertaker. 'What the bloody hell went wrong?' He shot down the stairs with the assistant at his heels. There was no sign of the monkey following them.

Aghast, I dashed to the door of the room from which they had fled and slammed it shut. I listened breathlessly. The monkey had stopped its noise on entering the place where his master lay. Corpse and monkey – I couldn't hear a peep out of either of them. I loaded another syringe back at the car, where the undertaker and his mate were standing on the pavement, nervously puffing at cigarettes. 'Get it right this time, friend,' said Mr Sowerberry lugubriously. 'Damn' right,' added Claypole.

There was still no sound when I returned to the landing for the third time. I threw open the door and stood back. Nothing came out. Cautiously, ever so cautiously, with the barrel of the gun poised like a metal extension to my nose, I put my head round the door. It was the Professor's bedroom. A brass bedstead with yellowing sheets, a marble wash-stand with porcelain ewer, a side-table stacked high with old copies of *The Lancet* and a heavy mahogany wardrobe. At the foot of the bed on a trestle lay a coffin. In the coffin was stretched the body of an old man, his face blue-grey above a long linen shift. Sitting on the corpse's ankles and blinking indifferently at me was the macaque. Very gently, with two fingers, he stroked his master's cold knees. All anger and fear had vanished from the animal's face. I raised the gun and fired. The dart hit him in the thigh. he gave a whimper, snatched briefly at the embedded dart and then quickly returned to stroking the corpse. Ten seconds later he collasped without any fuss and I went over and lifted him out of the coffin. *Requiescat in pace*, I thought – both of you.

The macaque was in a terrible condition, with a tumour in

the eye socket, vitamin deficiencies, a hernia, tooth and gum disease. He was also very old. There was nothing to be done for him and no-one who would want him. I injected him with an overdose of barbiturate.

Before I left the house I went into the room where the macaque had been living. It was an appalling sight. What had once been a bedroom was in utter ruin. A bed stripped to the springs, a cupboard torn to pieces, wallpaper shredded and plaster ulcerous with gaping holes, a dressing table with its mirror gone and covered with dusty shards of glass and years, not just days, of excrement and filth. Bits of wood, rusty metal and food – dried, decayed, mouldy and maggot-ridden – were strewn everywhere. I had never seen nor smelled so foul a habitation. It could not have been cleaned in a quarter of a century. Why a learned medical man should keep an animal like that for so long I will never understand. He probably loved it. It loved him, I am sure. But. . . . The answers are buried with both of them.

When I walked out of the house carrying the body of the macaque, the undertakers backed off. 'God, what a bleeding monster!' exclaimed the undertaker, wrinkling his nose.

'Serve it bloody well right,' opined the assistant.

They were both utterly wrong – and I felt curiously sad about the whole business.

4 Kim the Killer

The plump little old lady was dressed in the habit of a French nun from about 1880 – completely in black from the tip of her bonnet to the toes of her well-worn button boots. She smelled faintly of soap, pot-pourri and mothballs as she stood, hands clasped and lips moving soundlessly, before the faded sepia photograph of a glowering man in a monk's habit who could have been Rasputin's double. Her eyes were fixed unblinkingly on those of the man. Behind the old lady was a writing desk on which lay another photograph, perhaps one hundred years more recent than that of the mad monk's lookalike. It was a glossy, six-by-eight print of a bull killer whale caught in the instant when his three-ton body, caparisoned in a filigree of gleaming water-beads, reached the zenith of a great and joyous leap.

The little old lady (I never knew her full name but had been instructed to address her simply as 'La Soeur') finished her contemplation and turned towards me. A sweet smile – I was instantly reminded of the Queen Mother – lit up her face. 'All is going to be well,' she said in French.

I experienced (and my companions likewise, I was to learn later) an unmistakable sensation of relief, almost the first flickering of euphoria. 'What is the cause of all our troubles?' I asked.

La Soeur seemed to be searching for the right word. 'I am not medically qualified. This is not my rightful area, you understand.'

'But can you tell us anything?'

'Yes.' She glanced again towards the bearded man on the

wall. 'Father Antoine says there is a blockage – a grille – between the stomach and the intestines.'

'What kind of grille?'

'That I cannot say. Only that it is certain to cause death if it is not eliminated.'

'How do we do that?' Then, unreally, I heard myself add, 'Does the Father say anything about the treatment?'

La Soeur took my hand gently and gave a consoling squeeze. 'I am sorry, no. You do understand, don't you, that, well, whales are not *comme d'habitude* in our spiritual work here.'

'Of course, Sister. You have been very kind. So that is all we, you, can say?'

Abruptly the old lady wheeled round on her heels as if summoned back by the saturnine character in the photogravure. For a minute she resumed her attitude of rapt attention, staring up into his glaring eyes. Then she once more faced me. 'I have one more thing that the Father tells us,' she said. 'The whale will be made well by *you* – he feels *you* are the only person who can do it.' She pointed a pale finger at my head. 'It will happen in two hours' time and you will use three things!' La Soeur turned the palms of both hands outwards and shrugged her shoulders. 'I can do no more, Monsieur.'

We thanked her, gave her an envelope stuffed with francs, as we had been instructed, and went out into the world again with its bright, May-morning sunshine, the smell of Gitanes and croissants and washed pavements and bars with doors and windows being given an airing before the first pastis-drinkers arrived. I felt mentally shell-shocked, but also unexpectedly happy. Maybe everything was going to be all right.

We must have driven halfway back to Antibes, each of us deeply engrossed in our thoughts, before Michael Riddell said, 'Well, what do you make of that? A grille, two hours and then the use of three things. Is there anything like a grille – in an anatomical sense?'

'Not really,' I replied. 'I suppose you could say that a valve between the stomach and the duodenum, like the pyloric valve, is a grille. Or possibly the sphincter at the bottom end of the bile duct.'

'So what are you going to do, David?'

I stared for some time at the sea breaking gently on the pebbly shore beyond the railway line as we approached Marineland Côte d'Azur, where Michael was the director. 'I think,' I said eventually, 'I'll go to my room in the Tananarive at eleven o'clock, the time she indicated, and wait for inspiration about the three things.'

Anyone else but Michael would have laughed their heads off or driven me straight round to the nearest psycho-analyst. But 'Good idea,' he replied quietly. 'Somehow I *know* we're going to save the whale now.'

Lying on my bed in the Hotel Tananarive with the thunder of the coast-road traffic outside my window, I vainly tried to prepare my mind to be an empty vessel ready for filling with whatever esoteric pearls eleven o'clock might bring. It was impossible to turn myself into an instant adept in whatever mysteries the cult of La Soeur did business. Doubts and despair crowded in. So it had come to this, I thought. Having apparently exhausted the orthodox armoury of marine mammal medicine, I had agreed at least to listen to the little old lady whose reputation as a seer in the Côte d'Azur was apparently second to none. But beyond this lay – what? Shaking the bones, casting the runes or perhaps, more appropriately for a vet, prognosticating upon a chicken's entrails? Black magic, white magic? What would the Royal College of Veterinary Surgeons make of this dabbling?

I was, as they say in my native Lancashire, flummoxed. Kim, the biggest and most spectacular killer whale in any marineland outside the USA was ill, very ill, and steadily worsening. Caught in Icelandic waters, Kim might not have been absolutely A1 at Lloyd's when he first saw his captors as he was hauled out of the icy grey waters in November 1976. He had been the last animal caught that year. With hindsight, the grizzled, snuff-sniffing fishermen who had artfully encircled him with three miles of herring net and then slowly reduced the circle until French frogmen could jump in and fit a padded sling around the whale's body and hook it up to a crane that winched him onto the pitching deck, these whale-hunters who lived for weeks at sea on boiled sheep heads, strips of dried haddock and raw blubber, had noticed how unusually unresisting the bull whale had seemed.

Without any natural enemies, killer whales could, if they were so minded, literally run rings round the men in boats. Equipped as they are with twelve conical snapping teeth that may be five inches long on each jaw and great tails that can flail wickedly or power them through the seas at up to sixty miles per hour, they could blast their way through nets made of anything less robust than stainless steel. But they generally choose not to do so. Their sonar systems pick up the flimsy net cast in a wide sweep around them while they are busy feeding among the autumn run of herring. As the boats pull in the nets, thereby reducing the circumference of the circle, the whales keep their distance from the approaching curtain. Slowly they move to the centre of the ring. Is it trust, greed, carefree confidence in their own abilities or stupidity that makes them continue feeding, one eye on the advancing vessels, and with rarely any sign of fear? When the nets are brought up underneath them and the frogmen with the slings plop into the water, there is no sudden panic, no snapping at the limbs of the puny humans who lay hands on them – only perhaps a few pig-like squeals of mild apprehension through their blow holes. Once in the slings, as the greasing of the skin with a mixture of vaseline and lanolin begins in order to protect it during the voyage back to harbour, the animal may wriggle and flap its tail occasionally. A tiger, a gorilla, even a deer in a comparable situation wouldn't let its captors off so lightly.

Kim, however, had been unusually docile even for a killer whale. Maybe he had been already ailing when he cruised the Arctic seas that summer with the sun never setting while he and his school of perhaps five or six hundred fellows hunted walrus and seal off the Greenland coast, sounded deep to await the rising of the even deeper-diving fin and right whales with their bulky tongues (such delicacies for the taking) and tracked the shimmering shoals of numberless herring across the latitudes. Maybe. Certainly in his new home at Antibes, swimming with his mate Betty in the biggest pool in Europe, Kim seemed to be in the best of health. He grew, fattened, frolicked and learned quickly a wide repertoire of tricks. He appeared to prosper on a diet of finest Cornish mackerel and Scottish herring, supplemented each day with a hundred or so specially manufactured vitamin and mineral tables.

Andrew Greenwood and I monitored Kim regularly, just as we do all the other whales under our care. The key to preventive medicine in whales (as well as in dolphins and porpoises) is the laboratory analysis of blood samples. First, of course, catch your drop of blood – not as easily done as in a cow or a human being. I had tried taking blood from killer whales underwater on several occasions, scuba diving beneath their tails while armed with small vacuum tubes and needles. Not a chance – one prick of the needle and the great fluke had invariably flailed, not in anger but rather as a horse's tail whisks a bothersome fly from its hindquarters. In an explosion of foam, the whale, my sampling equipment and I had instantaneously parted company. Occasionally very large whales in the open ocean have permitted venous sampling in this way. The response to needle pricks seems to be related to the size of the beast. Smaller whales such as killers won't tolerate the free-swimming approach but can easily be trained to lift their tails out of the water for extraction of the necessary ten or twenty cc's of blood. The smallest whales, dolphins and porpoises, no matter how well-trained, will never go even so far and have to be caught and restrained for sampling or have their pools drained down.

Every month, Andrew or I would fly down to Antibes and between shows or at the end of the day Martin Padley, the chief trainer and an old friend, would give Kim the signal to roll over on his back and present the white undersurface of his tail flukes on the edge of the training platform. Although the whale could happily lie in this upside-down position for many minutes if necessary, it didn't take more than a few seconds to locate the specially designed blood vessels (they are built rather like man-made heat-exchanger tubes and allow the tail to act as an adjustable radiator in these marine mammals). One quick sting of the needle and the vacuum tube did the rest.

One day in 1980, the analysing machine in the laboratory at Newmarket where Kim's blood was sent for examination began to spew out a bizarre list of numbers. Andrew and I discussed the curious abnormalities. Among the most worrying was an unusually high level of protein. Detailed laboratory tests showed that all the excess protein was in the form of immune antibodies. Kim's body, this meant, was fighting something somewhere in his insides. Yet he looked as fit as a fiddle.

We took more samples and again found the high level of antibodies. At the time it seemed tempting to suppose that perhaps there was nothing amiss. Our maximum and minimum levels of normality for many tests on exotic animals are still being constantly modified in the light of experience. Perhaps Kim had recovered from a severe illness in his childhood that left him carrying lots of protective immunity – but I was sure that such explanations were wrong. Week after week in Newmarket and later in Nice when a hospital laboratory generously volunteered to run a parallel series of tests, the electronic machines hummed and whirled and computed and disgorged strips of graph paper. It was always the same: too much protein. And the level was slowly but steadily rising. I checked and double-checked all the information I could glean by prodding, probing, sampling and testing Kim, usually working at night under the light of arc lamps. It was cooler then, so there was less chance of overheating. With their pool drained of water, the two whales would grumpily lie

60

stranded on the bottom, he producing thunderclaps as he beat his broad tail menacingly on the fibreglass pool lining and she snapping at our legs if we walked too close to her head.

Every possible diagnostic examination was carried out, but still we found ourselves no closer. I was convinced that there was a sizeable centre of infection somewhere that was at the root of the problem, but the tests for liver, kidney and other organ function were normal. There was no indication of where the trouble lay. Oh to be a human doctor! 'Lie down on the couch, please. Does it hurt here? Can you say "augh"? – Touch the tip of your toes if you can. Ever had a dizzy spell?' Even an ordinary vet dealing with domestic and farm animals has it easier. A killer whale like Kim can be up to thirty feet in length and weigh ten tons. His hydrodynamically-shaped body is tightly encased in hard blubber, overlaid with skin as smooth as a billiard ball. No pulse to feel with one's fingers. A massive girth in which x-rays from the usual portable machines get hopelessly lost. Organs that may lie three feet deep, well away from the physician's enquiring hands. No knees to jerk obligingly when tapped by the rubber hammer. And how to get a glimpse of the tonsils or even the eye if the animal decides to keep everything tightly shut?

I was anxious to look inside Kim's stomach with a fibre-optic gastroscope if possible. Maybe there was a grumbling ulcer. The instrument we normally use for such internal examinations is the longest made – 1.6 metres, and originally designed for looking up into human colons from the rear end – but it was nowhere near long enough. Even using it on Betty, I could only get a glimpse of the first part of the stomach just at the bottom of the gullet. Michael Riddell suggested obtaining an industrial fibre-optic viewing device, of the type used for remote inspection of furnaces, jet engines and so on. They come up to four metres long but, of course, don't carry the sophisticated lens-washing, air-blowing and instrument-carrying channels that are found on the medical instruments. Also, they are constructed in one long, inflexible metal tube and cannot move round and explore like my gastroscope which can literally be guided through all the corners and into every nook and cranny of the oesophagus, stomach, duodenum and intestines, or if necessary the windpipe.

I decided to try Michael's idea, though, and Citroën in Paris readily agreed to lend an industrial fibre-optic to us. Guy, the clerk of works at the marineland, modified the tube by strapping to it an air-line for inflation of the stomach to provide better viewing, a water-tube and spray to wash the lens on the tip of the instrument and an ingenious pair of pincer jaws just in case I felt like grabbing hold of something I found. Although broader in diameter than my gastroscope, this ersatz Heath Robinson version would have no trouble passing down Kim's gullet. These whales possess broad and elastic oesophaguses and can easily swallow whole seals. The stomach of one killer dissected in Denmark in 1862 was found to contain thirteen dolphins and fourteen seals with another seal still in its throat. What I feared was that the inflexibility of the rigid tube would be a problem in restricting the field of view. We would also have to be very careful not to damage the animal if he wriggled while the instrument was inside him. I had ruled out sedation save for a small shot of librium – gastroscopy isn't painful and I didn't want to depress his breathing while he was stranded out of water. On dry land big whales run a risk of lung problems at the best of times.

When, around midnight on the night I had selected for the operation, Kim was lying high and dry under the stars with Martin wetting down his skin from time to time with cold water, my helpers in their wet suits standing by and the gastroscope attached to its powerful light source, I gave the word for the mouth to be opened.

Years earlier, Martin and I had found that first Cuddles, the Flamingo Park whale, and then Calypso, the big female we brought from Canada via Cleethorpes to Nice, didn't care to open their jaws for dental inspection, force-feeding or other such indignities. Against muscles capable of exerting thousands of pounds of pressure per square inch, there wasn't much point in applying the standard techniques that work so well with dogs, cattle and horses. And with teeth such as a whale's a chance bite would have meant amputation at the wrist rather than a mere painful bitten finger. So it is always essential to insert a gag in the shape of a beam of wood between the jaws before doing anything inside a whale, but how to get the gag in through the interlocking barricades of fearsome teeth? All attempts to get a mere crack open by careful use of a padded crowbar, steel jemmies and wedges of teak had proved futile. I had even considered numbing the jaw with local anaesthetic and extracting a tooth or two in order to create a suitable portal of entry when Martin, as he kept the whales wet with a hosepipe of fresh water, found by chance that playing the jet of water lightly onto the teeth and gums and 'tickling' them would cause the animals to open their jaws briefly. The wooden gag could then be quickly slipped into place and held at each end by men who were instructed to move with the beam if the whale swung its head about but on pain of death not to let go. I had seen the effects in the USA of what happened to a gag which slipped from the grip of its handlers: the powerful stubby tongue of the whale spat the offending object out as easily as if it were a matchstick and, as the beam of wood was ejected whilst the whale was swinging its head sideways, the gag clouted one assistant squarely on the face, knocking him out cold and breaking his nose. Meanwhile the jaws had closed on the arm of the vet who had not been quite quick enough in removing it. His mangled wrist required extensive plastic surgery.

Now we had constructed a long, four-inch-square beam of wood to use as a gag for Kim, with rope loops at each end for the men to hang on to. In the centre of the beam a slot had been cut through which I intended to slide the gastroscope. Martin turned on a hose and played the water on Kim's lips. The assistants crowded ready to jam the gag into the gap as soon as it appeared. The water splashed against the tight black slit of

Kim's mouth and streamed in rivulets off his chin. The trap that could behead a polar bear stayed shut. Martin increased the water pressure. Kim swivelled one dark eye at him and blew a jet of warm air, friendly as a cow's breath, but there still wasn't room to slip so much as a razor blade between the lips. Boom! Kim slowly raised his tail and then slammed it down onto the pool bottom. The ground shook. The fibreglass of the pool lining hummed. Kim was growing impatient. The great mouth (or was it just my imagination?) tightened even more and stayed shut. More water. More pressure. Boom! Boom! The tail crashed down again and began to steam. Kim's impatience was ripening into anger. 'Put on full pressure and get in closer,' I said. Martin directed the jet at point-blank range straight onto the tip of Kim's snout. The big whale didn't unclench his teeth one micron. Most definitely, though, he did finally run out of patience with the landlubbers gathered around him.

A whale out of water with no limbs to give it purchase and several tons of weight resting on its breastbone is not as helpless as one might suppose. The mighty muscles of the back all converge to power the tail and, as well as moving the flukes up and down, they can pull sideways into the bargain. Kim brought his lumbar muscles into play and slashed his tail fiercely to the left. One man who was standing a bit too close was swept cleanly off his feet and thrown sprawling with a dislocated knee. The tail reached the limit of its sideways travel and then scythed to the right. It didn't connect with anyone this time but its impetus swung Kim's trunk askew. He began to curve and uncurve the length of his body, squirming on the damp plastic like a giant tadpole. His mouth stayed clam-tight. Jumping out of his way, we tried to keep our distance. Another man lost his footing and slipped. Kim twisted and squirmed his glistening bulk towards the fellow as he was scrambling to his feet and caught him in the solar plexus with a killer whale karate chop. The bull killer gave a squeal of victory and cracked two of the man's ribs for good measure with another flick of the fluke.

'Everybody out!' My shout signalled the end of our attempt to look down Kim's throat. We retreated with our wounded and defeated, opened the valves to refill the whale pool. If there was anything in Kim's stomach, we weren't going to find out that way.

With Kim proving a rather unco-operative patient except for his tolerance of blood sampling, diagnosis was largely dependent on information provided by the laboratory tests. Microbiological studies of the air from his lungs could be done by holding a glass plate containing bacterial culture medium in gelatine upside down over his blow hole and waiting for him to exhale. Stool analysis was also possible, though collecting the stool of whales is the ultimate in water sports. The droppings of killer whales, indeed of any marine mammal, are elusive, ephemeral things and their collection demands dedication, a delicate touch and the ability to keep one's mouth shut. Consider the problem: whales' droppings are normally of liquid consistency and bottle-green in colour. The liquid is emitted in pretty little clouds of bottle-green from time to time and completely unpredictably. Once on the outside, it rapidly dissolves into the sea water and effectively disappears.

So you fancy yourself as a killer whale stool hunter? OK – arm yourself with a sampling vessel, something wide-mouthed like an old jam-jar, and present yourself at the edge of the pool. Problem one is seeing that bottle-green cloud in what is often bottle-green water. If it is released while the whale is moving at speed you certainly won't get a chance to see it at all. But suppose you, jam-jar clasped in your enthusiastic stool-hunter's palm, are lucky enough to spot the cloud puffing out from the whale as it naps peacefully in the water. Then, intrepid stool person, you must strike at once – there is not a moment to lose!

Slipping smoothly into the water, you must paddle over to the whale and dive down *into* the bottle-green goodies, jam-jar held forward like a cavalryman's sabre. This is where your long and gruelling training comes to fruition. Your aim is to scoop some of the already partially-dispersed gunge into your jar. This is where you are apt to encounter problems two through ninety-nine, as the Americans would say. The whale, dozing and dreaming whale dreams, is never asleep in the same way that we humans recline in the arms of Morpheus. One side of a whale's brain sleeps at a time while the other side keeps watch for things like humans or other curiosities that might drop in. As the whale moves to see what you are up to and as you do your quickest but at the same time, you hope, smoothest dog-paddle in the direction of your quarry, your combined movements swirl and twirl the water and in a flash the bottle-green gubbins is gone. Even if you are lucky enough to be hanging around a whale's rear end on the off-chance, as it were, when the world around you suddenly goes the colour of crème de menthe, there is a snag with jam-jars under water: they are already full, and you can't put a quart into a pint pot. Sweep the jar through the cloud as it swirls round your ears and then take it up to the surface for a look. The clear water in the jar will show that your prey got away. So next time try flailing your jar with abandon – and you will find that the turbulence you create simply disperses the cloud even more certainly.

Some old hands try stalking the whale's fundamental orifice. This is the virtuoso's game and not one for beginners. It means sitting under a whale's bottom, obviously in scuba gear, waiting for him to feel the urge to relieve himself. It is oh so easy to fall asleep down there, waiting and waiting in sun-dappled water, or to have the whale, just for fun, chew through your air-supply pipes or, if in one's enthusiasm one touches the animal's anal region with the jar, to receive a fierce blow from a down-beat of the tail flukes as a warning not to be too familiar. Whale droppings, which can yield information on disorders of digestion, the presence of microbes, parasites or toxins or of bleeding in the gastro-intestinal tract are

66

like gold-dust to the whale doctor – and nearly as difficult to obtain.

In the end, no matter how we juggled the figures and pondered over what information I did manage to squeeze out of Kim, both Andrew and I came back again and again to the worrying conclusion that there was a nest of infection somewhere in the big whale, but we had no idea where it was. To watch him feed and play and roar round the whale pool, no-one would possibly have imagined our misgivings. I decided to aim blindfold by giving Kim a course of antibiotics and seeing what that did to the antibody proteins. Accordingly, one hundred capsules of the drug were secreted in his herring three times a day. The protein level stayed high and the antibiotic course had barely finished when the time came for me to issue the health certificate which the insurance underwriters at Lloyd's of London required. Like most of his kind in captivity, Kim was insured for around £300,000. With such large sums at stake I had to be scrupulously careful, and I informed Lloyd's of the problem and its possible cause. Their reaction was, as I had anticipated, postponement of the renewal of cover until I had a perfect blood sample. Kim was now uninsured but Michael, fighting to put the marineland back on its feet after several uncertain years, took it philosophically. 'Whatever it needs or costs to get him right, do it,' he said.

During the next few months I tried various lines of therapy – the latest anti-bacterial drugs, tissue-healing hormones and anti-inflammatory compounds. Nothing availed but still Kim remained apparently fit and certainly active. Until the beginning of 1981 when, one bright April morning, the nightwatchman of the marineland discovered a curious, spindle-shaped, orange object floating on the surface of the whale pool. He scooped it out with a shrimping net. It was the remains of a plastic beach ball, burst, deflated and folded into a multilayered miniature rugby football. It was as hard as iron, and adhering to it were shreds of partially digested fish.

Michael called me and reported the find. There was little doubt that it had been regurgitated by one of the whales, almost certainly Kim. The soft plastic of the ball had been vulcanised by the action of the powerful stomach acids. Beach balls were used in abundance during the whale shows when the animals 'played football', hitting the orange-coloured spheres high and far into the crowds of spectators. The latter were allowed to keep any balls that came their way and could perhaps have thrown one or two back, unseen by any of the staff, after the shows. Certainly none of the trainers had ever reported Kim or Betty swallowing a ball. But there it was – a foreign body that had obviously been inside a whale for a considerable time. Could it be the cause of my strange blood results?

I had grave doubts. The plastic 'spindle' had fairly pointed ends, but I couldn't imagine it doing much damage inside the capacious first stomach of a whale. Even dolphins, during experiments conducted by the US Navy, had happily carried telemetry devices the size of pint beer-cans lying free in their stomachs. Whales have even more space than dolphins and a tough stomach wall that can cope with a hundredweight of raw and spiky fish a time. I monitored the blood samples. No sign of the antibodies falling. A few days after the first ball was found, another was ejected, again in the deflated, rigid spindle form. Kim regurgitated it without any fuss under the eyes of the same watchman. Then the next night two further balls were returned, then another in mid-show some days later. Within the space of the following three weeks, fifteen identical balls, all folded into the neat rugger ball shape, were recovered. Surely these objects couldn't have been doing any good in Kim's innards? But still there was no sign of change, either in the laboratory tests or in the whale's behaviour. Inexorably the antibodies in his blood crept upwards. Where would it all end? The balls, I was convinced, were a red herring. There was something somewhere much more sinister and persistent.

More months passed and, apart from the continuing insidious rise in antibodies in his blood, all seemed well with the big whale. Then one autumn day he suddenly changed. His appetite waned and he didn't want to perform his tricks for Martin or play with Betty. I caught the next airbus down to Nice and once again went through the routine of draining the whale pool, giving Kim an overhaul and taking blood samples. By this time we had developed excellent systems of co-operation with another hospital laboratory not far from the Marineland Côte d'Azur. At no matter what time of day or night, the lab would process Kim's samples within a matter of minutes on the most up-to-date analysers. Blood was taken to the hospital by a skilful maniac on a motor-bike and results were telephoned to the marineland where Michael, his team and I waited to decide on therapy. Speed was essential with the heavy whale out of water, its weight pressing down on its lungs, and we gradually refined the process so that Kim was floating again less than an hour after we had first gone into the pool to collect the samples. Later we found it possible to locate blood vessels lying deep in the dorsal fin and then we eliminated beaching the whale completely, doing our sampling by paddling around Kim as he lay with just a few millimetres of water under his belly.

The antibodies were still high but there was now also something else. Increasing numbers of white blood cells signalled an active infection. With no indication as to what kind of infection I was facing or where it was, I had to choose drugs blind. I settled on amoxycillin, a new broad-spectrum synthetic penicillin. Now to inject it. The vet who injects killer whales has a little in common with the matador standing ready to plunge the *espada* into the waiting bull. The needles I use are eight, ten or even twelve inches long and they have to be placed smoothly through the skin and thick blubber into the muscles that run along the back. Wrongly placed, the drug may set up a progressive destruction of the blubber fat or at least not be efficiently absorbed. With the needle in place, giant syringes are attached and several whole bottles of the chosen drug are injected.

Kim responded well to the amoxycillin shots and within a few days seemed to be his old self again. The white cell count fell but, ominously, the antibodies stayed high. A few months later Kim fell ill again and responded to antibiotic therapy. Then there was a third attack after only a few weeks. I was growing moderately concerned. The more I thought about it, the more it seemed logical for there to be an abscess somewhere deep in the body; not in a vital organ except perhaps the lung, although his breathing was normal and his breath sweet. The likeliest site was in the space between the lungs or in the abdominal cavity. Pus in its centre, of which there must be a considerable amount, was causing the antibody rise and perhaps if there was a thick, gristly capsule to the abscess which stopped antibiotic penetration, that explained the recurrence of the attacks and the chronic nature of the underlying disease. I discussed it again with Andrew and we agreed that chronic abscess was Kim's problem. The attacks were, we reasoned, caused by bacteria advancing out of their walled abscess citadel and setting up acute feverish episodes.

Soon I found myself facing more frequent attacks and, even more worrying, ones which lasted longer. Worse still, the amoxycillin began to lose its effectiveness. I turned to other drugs and for a time seemed to regain the upper hand. But eventually it became clear that I was fighting an ever more desperate battle. I was having great difficulty reducing the white cell counts and I was troubled by signs that the antibiotic treatments were encouraging opportunist fungi to set up secondary problems. What was I to do? Was there any way of clinching the diagnosis? How could I locate the abscess if it existed? Could it be drained?

At the same time I was under pressure from friends and colleagues who questioned my reasoning as to the handling of the case. The laboratory doctors talked of cancer, the French vet considered Kim to be leukaemic, it was suggested that we were overtreating and causing more trouble than the original complaint, there were those who thought that stomach ulcers and the plastic balls were at the bottom of it all, and there were constant red herrings thrown into the ring by Kim himself who, for example, on several occasions gave positive test readings for the presence of brucellosis, a disease that causes abortion in cattle and undulant fever in man. This latter finding caused me to test other animals, including the guard dog and all the personnel, for evidence of brucellosis. We found none.

I stuck to the 'abscess in a place unknown' theory and received constant support and encouragement from Michael. He was the one who, as director, had to answer to the owner of the marineland, Comte Pauze d'Ivoire de la Poype, for all the bills – and at one stage we were spending £600 per day on special drugs. So it came about that, with the attacks becoming more and more frequent and severe, I eventually received a 'phone call from Comte de la Poype himself. He didn't beat about the bush. 'I know, my dear David,' he said, 'that you are doing your best, but I have a suggestion.'

Aha, I thought, I've treated whales that had orchestras hired to play to them while they were sick, seen the store of Bisquit brandy that Billy Smart swore was the only true medicine for sick elephants, tried acupuncture on an arthritic giraffe with some success and heard Mass said for a dying dolphin. What was M. le Comte going to come up with? I knew he was sometimes sceptical of orthodox medicine. Maybe it would be homoeopathy or some French country herbal remedy. So long as it isn't positively harmful and doesn't interfere with my approach, I'll try anything if I'm in a hole with a tough case. It keeps the owners happy and, well, you never know. The main thing is to *win*. What or who takes the credit is of no consequence. I was accustomed to spending weeks wrestling with a sick animal and then, if it finally recovered, hearing a keeper say something like, 'I'm sure it's the peppermint tea I gave it that made all the difference' or 'I knew it would be OK if I stuck a clove of garlic in its ear just like my old dad used to do.'

71

Matt Kelly, the old head keeper at Belle Vue Zoo in Manchester, had been a great one for that sort of thing: peeing on an antelope's food ('bound to make it eat') and adding raspberry leaf tea to a pregnant chimpanzee's drink 'to ensure an easy birth'.

The Frenchman continued. 'My suggestion is, well I know you may think it, 'ow you say, a little bizarre, but – er – I have arranged for you to have a meeting with an Antoiniste Sister tomorrow morning at nine o'clock in Nice.'

'Antoiniste Sister?'

'She is *fantastique* – a clairvoyant I think you would call her. She knows things in the most incredible way.' He went on to explain. The Antoinistes were a group which originated at the turn of the century following the writings of Louis Antoine, a Belgian miner. His teachings had Christian, pantheistic and theosophical elements, with particular stress on healing by laying on of hands. The Sister in Nice had a formidable reputation as a medium. He had secretly taken a photograph of Kim to the lady some days previously and she had diagnosed something wrong in the wall between the stomach and the intestine. What was more he had taken the photograph to another clairvoyant in Paris, the most famous in France and one employed regularly by M. Mitterrand and other important personages. The second clairvoyant amazingly had also looked at the photograph and without hesitation had said, 'There is something stuck in the wall between stomach and intestine.' Neither medium had been given any medical history and neither claimed to know anything about killer whales or veterinary medicine. 'So you see, maybe if you went to see La Soeur in Nice . . .'

M. le Comte's suggestions are never to be taken lightly. If he hadn't been deadly serious he wouldn't have been ringing me personally from Paris. 'Yes, of course I'll go,' I told him. 'I'll take Michael along. My French can cope with basic medical matters but isn't up to more esoteric subjects.'

'Good. She will be waiting for you in the chapel at nine.'

My travelling clock peeped to announce eleven o'clock. I waited for enlightenment. Three things, La Soeur had promised. A mixture of drugs? Three new lines of therapy? Three acupuncture points? My mind waited, not totally unconvinced, for the inspiration. Images of Kim, the remarkable little old nun and the figure three flickered across the black screen of my closed eyelids.

Nothing happened. The traffic continued to roar. The room maid's vacuum hummed in the corridor outside. For half an hour I lay relaxing and ready for the revelation. It was not to be. I rose and walked back to the marineland.

'Well?' Michael said, eyebrows raised, as I went into his office. 'What do we have to do?' 'I haven't a clue,' I replied.

Martin Padley burst in behind me. 'For God's sake come and look at Kim,' he gasped. 'I think he's gone blind!'

The three of us ran through the park to the whale pool. Kim was floating some yards away from the side, his head facing away from us. Martin took a handful of herrings from the fish bucket and threw them hard at the water a little in front of the whale's snout. They made a sharp splash and, as if wakened sharply from a reverie, Kim gave a start, opened his mouth and lunged at them. He missed them completely and they shimmered down past his flippers into the depths. The whale turned uncertainly in their direction and then I saw the nearest eye. It was snowy white. Kim turned full circle trying to locate the fish – living now in clear water, he had, like most cetaceans in captivity, stopped using his sonar echo-location devices. The other eye came into view. Its surface too was totally opaque. 'You're right, Martin,' I murmured in dismay, 'he can't see a thing.'

Hurriedly putting on a wet suit, I entered Kim's pool and paddled over to him. It was best to see the eyes close up under water. My fears were quickly confirmed: the white eyes weren't simple inflammations of the corneas but something much more serious. Infection was active deep in the interior of the eyes. The germs from the hidden source somewhere in his body had mounted a terrible guerilla raid.

'I must begin chloramphenicol injections into the eye straightaway,' I told Michael as I climbed out of the water. 'Things are looking bloody grim.' In twenty-five years of struggling with the myriad maladies of exotic animals, I don't think I have ever felt more down-hearted.

5 In the Palace of the Sheik

The Bedou guard raised his Armalite rifle and pointed it at my head. He looked like a pint-sized Omar Sharif, except that his teeth were stained brown and he smelled of onions. His originally curious expression had hardened suddenly to one of tense suspicion. Fixing me with brittle black eyes, he called out in alarm in staccato Arabic and other men came running. I stood still, clutching the object that I had just uncovered for his inspection at the sentry post and which had produced his threatening reaction. It was an expensive binocular microscope.

The Sheik's palace guards surrounded me and my companion Dr Qassan, a Lebanese ornithologist, and all stared at the double-barrelled instrument with its shining wheels, condenser, diaphragm and light source. One Bedou, in a cream-coloured dish-dash with crossed bandoliers of copper-jacketed bullets and a curved Arab dagger in a chased silver scabbard behind his belt, reached out and took the microscope from my hands. 'What's up?' I murmured to Qassan, feeling suddenly a little uneasy.

'The microscope – they don't know what it is. It looks like a gun to them.' He began to explain to them and showed them how the eyepiece is removed and the lens-turret revolved. But without the eyepieces the microscope's twin tubes did look rather like a double barrel, and the clicking turret just might have been some sort of magazine, and the heavy stand did fit comfortably into the Bedou's shoulder when he tried it, making a passable butt.

'What's the Arabic for microscope?' I asked.

'*Microscope*. But they've never heard of, let alone seen, such a thing.'

It took another twenty minutes of fast talking by Qassan, with me stripping down the microscope into its component parts, before we were allowed to enter the palace grounds with the suspect piece of equipment, cleared of being possible Mossad or PLO assassins.

Sheik Jamal's palace, a pastel pink and green complex of single-storey buildings in a garden of palms and tamarisks surrounded by a high wall, is just one of half a dozen such residences that he possesses in the oasis town of Al Ain. In other parts of the Arab Emirates he has as many again and he travels constantly between them, spending perhaps only days or sometimes a few hours in any one place. Like all the sheiks, he is highly security-minded and moves in a haphazard and unpredictable fashion, often without more than a few minutes warning to his entourage. And where he goes, there go his favourite falcons, ready for a messenger to ride in from the deep desert with news of stone curlew or bustard for the hunting. To visit him and talk falcons I might have to travel five or five hundred miles, and when he sent for me it was politic to go – at once. In the Gulf a sheik's command still overrides all other matters save perhaps the recent decease of the commanded one, and falcons take precedence over men. Often I have been ushered straight into the presence of a sheik who wanted to show me a peregrine with a sore eye or a saker falcon with catarrh, while the ambassador of some great state was kept waiting in an ante-room, perhaps for an hour or two. For the Bedou nobleman the traditional love of hawking, of tracking wily birds over an inconstant sea of sand, of comprehending wind and sky and the movement of shadows, and of the ancient arts of barbaric surgery and arcane medicine for birds of prey, is more important than the flummery of visiting congressmen, trade missions and Euro-MPs.

On this particular day Dr Qassan, the bird curator at Al Ain

Zoo and an authority on the bird life of the Gulf, had tracked down Sheik Jamal to the pink and green palace and sent a messenger with request for an audience. I was on one of my regular visits to the Emirates to discuss things with Chris Furley, and had important information concerning an outbreak of lung disease in some of the sheik's peregrines. I needed urgently to explain the situation to His Excellency himself. Back had come the word that we should go at once. The lung disease, common among falcons in Arabia, was *radad*, an infection caused by the aspergillus fungus. During a recent visit to Al Ain, Andrew Greenwood had taken cultures of the straw-lined walls of one of the sheik's new falcon houses. The straw was part of an ingenious, cheap air conditioning system developed in Israel and copied by the Arabs. A cistern on top of the house supplied water which trickled down over the straw. Air blowing through the gaps in the straw was thus automatically cooled by evaporation, producing a pleasant environment inside which was ideal for the hawks even during the hottest days of summer.

Unfortunately, damp straw also produces an ideal environment for the growth of moulds. Andrew had grown exactly the same fungus from the wall as we had found in dead falcons' lungs. My purpose now was to explain this to the Sheik, show him the evidence and propose either the tearing down of the new falcon house or perpetual disinfection of the straw. As well as the microscope I was carrying with me some stained slides of the fungus germs, taken from both the straw and the birds' lungs, and a culture dish of jelly medium showing to the naked eye large colonies of fungus radiating out from a piece of unmistakable straw. I knew from bitter experience that simply saying things to the Arabs through an interpreter wasn't enough, particularly where falcons were concerned. They considered themselves experts in all hawking matters by birthright. Non-Bedous, particularly non-Arab foreigners such as myself, were doubtfully regarded, no matter how illustrious their qualifications. I had to make the case stark and simple and, if I could, visible.

After negotiating the guards, we entered one of the palace buildings and were shown into a garish room badly hung with expensive pink wallpaper and lit by batteries of fluorescent tubes. In the middle of the room a large square of yellow plastic sheet had been spread on the thick pile carpet. The Sheik, a burly, pale-skinned individual of about thirty with black beard and moustache, lounged with his cronies on sofas placed around three sides of the room with hawks here and there sitting on gloved fists or cushions beside the men. All rose when we entered and we made the rounds, shaking hands and chanting the familiar Arabic greeting, 'Salaam aleikum'. I was motioned to a place on the Sheik's right hand. Qassan sat next to me. Servants entered with metal trays bearing roast haunches of lamb, spiced rice and red jelly and put them on the plastic sheet. Everyone got down on their haunches and began to tuck into the food with enthusiasm. Breaking off pieces of meat from the joints and then eating it using only the right hand wasn't difficult, but scooping up soggy rice and shaping it into a compact mouthful with nothing more than five fingers was trickier. The Bedou did it fast and neatly, rarely leaving a grain of rice stuck to their beards. I made a fearful mess of my face and the carpet around me. The Arabs raced through the meal, gobbling down palmfuls of jelly after the lamb and washing all down, when the trays were empty, with cups of cold water. I finished last, having consumed little because of my clumsiness and feeling like a toddler in dire need of bib, high chair, pusher and spoon. Then we all trooped off to wash in an adjoining bathroom after which we again assembled in the pink room.

'So, Doctor, how are you?' asked the Sheik, with Qassan interpreting.

'Well, your Excellency, and happy to be back in Arabia.'

'So, Doctor, how are you?' Same question. In polite Arabic

78

the opening remark is repeated three or four times and each time answered with a different elaborate pleasantry. In English it sounds odd – as if one's questioner were deaf or inattentive. I had to answer politely, 'It is wet again in London, your Excellency.'

'So, Doctor, how are you?'

'I have had a trouble-free journey and will be here another seven days.'

'So, Doctor, how are you?'

'I am pleased to bring news of your Excellency's falcons.'

Opening formalities over, I went straight in to the matter of the falcon disease. 'We have found the cause of the *radad* in your birds, sir.'

'Ah, yes, the *radad*. Caused by feeding bad meat followed by good meat.' The Sheik gave a signal and a servant began to move round with tiny cups and a pot of cardamom coffee.

'Well, perhaps,' I said diplomatically, 'but at the root of it is a mould, a sort of mushroom that grows in the lung.'

The Sheik sniffed and sipped his coffee. He didn't seem to have heard me.

'And we have found the same mushroom growing in the walls of the new falcon house.'

'So, Doctor?' No doubt about it – he was unimpressed.

'The falcon house is dangerous, your Excellency.'

'Dangerous?' Now he was becoming positively indignant.

'Yes, sir. The birds catch the mushroom from the straw in the walls.'

'*Radad* is caused by good meat fed after bad meat, Doctor.'

'But there is a germ, sir, like there is a germ that causes boils or tuberculosis.'

The Sheik looked at me and gave an indulgent smile. 'Boils come from sexual frustration – a melancholia of men deprived of the company of women. And tuberculosis is from transgressing the law of the Prophet, all honour be upon him, and eating the meat of pigs.' He uttered the words with confident finality.

'We have seen the mushrooms in the lungs and we have seen

the same mushrooms in the straw, your Excellency. I have brought specimens and a microscope for you to see for yourself.'

Sheik Jamal let a string of jade worry-beads trickle through his fingers and suddenly looked interested. 'You have brought something to show me?'

'Yes, sir – I can show you *radad* in action.'

Qassan plugged the microscope into a power socket and set it up on the arm of the Sheik's couch. I laid out my specimens. Taking the lid off the jelly medium, I pointed out the fragment of straw and the fuzzy circles of greyish-black mould growing from it. 'That is the trouble with the falcon house,' I said.

Sheik Jamal clapped his hands. 'Send for Mahmoud!' he told the servant who appeared. Very shortly a squat, balding Arab in European dress came into the room and paid his respects to the assembled company. I noticed he eyed me with sour distaste as he touched my fingers and murmured, 'Salaam aleikum.'

'This is Mr Mahmoud, my engineer from Cairo,' said the Sheik. 'He built the new falcon house.' Addressing the Egyptian, he continued, 'Dr Taylor here says the new house is killing the falcons. What do you say to that?'

The tubby little engineer wagged a sweating brow and gesticulated dramatically. 'Is nonsense,' he said in English. 'Cannot be. Why you say that, Doctor?'

'Because I have found *radad* fungus in the straw!' I pointed to the microscope.

'Pshaw!' The Egyptian tossed his head and went on in rapid Arabic, pulling a small philatelist's magnifying glass out of his shirt pocket. He flourished the glass in front of the Sheik and pointed at me from time to time.

'He is saying that he also has inspected the straw,' whispered Qassan, 'with his magnifier.'

'Inspected?' I choked under my breath. 'That toy can magnify about times two. It's only for looking at details on postage stamps!'

'Doctor.' It was the Sheik again. 'Mr Mahmoud is quite confident that there is nothing wrong with the building.'

'Nothing wrong with the building,' I agreed. 'The straw just happens to be infected. Mr Mahmoud couldn't have been expected to know about *radad*.'

Severely the Sheik wagged a finger at me. 'Mr Mahmoud says he knows all about *radad*, Doctor, and he says there must be another cause.'

The engineer, sweating copiously by now, was sitting glaring at me with an air of injured dignity. I switched on the microscope light and slipped a slide of the fungus in a falcon's lung under the objective lens. I adjusted the illumination, searched for a typical area of infection and with the wheels quickly brought it into focus. Coloured in shades of bright blue by the biological stain, the densely packed strands of fungus with dark spores on their ends looked exactly like a thicket of trees – a fantastic forest in aquamarine. 'Your Excellency, please look down there.'

The Sheik squinted down the twin tubes. His eyes widened. 'Ayee,' he whispered quietly. 'I see . . . I see . . . TREES!'

'Yes,' I said triumphantly, 'and that is the mould – the mushroom, the fungus, aspergillus, *radad* – in the lung of your falcon.'

Sheik Jamal looked up and then turned to an old Bedou with a face like a pickled walnut sitting in a corner wearing a rather grimy robe and stroking a hooded saker falcon's neck with one leathery brown finger. He was the Sheik's chief falconer. 'O, Saeed,' said the Sheik, addressing the old man, 'come and see. Tell me what you think of this. The Doctor has found it growing inside Akhbar the peregrine.'

Saeed the falconer rose and came over to the microscope. With eyes that could read in soft dune sand how long ago the faint footprints of a houbara had been made and that could watch the stoop of a distant hawk in what to other men was but shimmering white, empty air, Saeed looked for the first time in his life into another world. He stared hard for a moment and then straightened up. '*Ashjaar!*' he exclaimed. '*Ashjaar! Ashjaar!*' Looking at his Sheik, he began to laugh – a deep, hearty belly laugh. In between guffaws he spoke in Bedou Arabic that Qassan had difficulty in understanding. The other men in the room now also began to laugh and the Sheik joined in.

'What is the cause of Saeed's amusement?' I asked the Sheik when the mirth began to subside.

'Saeed speaks but the truth,' he replied. 'He says your machine shows *ashjaar* – trees. But how can trees grow inside a bird? Big bird or small trees?' Everyone except Qassan and me began to chuckle again.

'Trees inside a bird! What nonsense is this?' the engineer said, taking the opportunity to add his two penn'orth.

I had to my astonishment lost credibility by my show of modern laboratory technique. Perhaps, I thought, it was only to be expected – to a man who has never seen such a thing before, a microscope does need some explanation. It really is a window into another, invisible world. 'Your Excellency,' I said, now going for broke, 'to get back to the *radad* – I have two marvellous new remedies.' Perhaps the straightforward, horse-doctor-with-magic-potion approach was all that was necessary. 'Firstly I would like you to add a special powder to the water in the falcon house cistern. It will keep *radad* away.' Actually it was a non-toxic anti-fungal disinfectant that would sterilise the straw as it trickled down. 'Secondly I have some tablets here for any more sick birds.' This was ketoconazole, the new anti-fungal drug.

Sheik Jamal at least listened to what I had to say and inspected the tablets I produced from my bag. 'Thank you, Doctor,' he said. 'I am honoured that such an expert doctor should come to discuss my falcons and give me such valuable advice.' He rose – it was the end of my audience. 'We will use the tablets, if you are certain they will not cause tiredness or loss of virility or weakness or lack of stamina in the hawks.'

'Your Excellency, they will do nothing but good, I assure you,' I said as I went round shaking hands.

The tablets were never used and the powder disinfectant, the only one of its kind in the world, is unfortunately manufactured by a company with the name of Goldschmidt and so is as unimportable into that Arab country as pork chops pickled in brandy. The magnifying glass of engineer Mahmoud continues to find no evidence of mould or mushrooms, let alone trees, in the straw walls of the falcon house. The Sheik's falcons continue to live in the straw house and they continue to die from *radad*. But Qassan tells me that Saeed, the old falconer, is working on it: he bathes the chest of ailing birds with fermented date pulp. After all, he says, if they die it is Kismet, the will of Allah – quite a different matter from being killed by Ingleesi Doctor's new-fangled nostrums.

In Arabia I had become accustomed to peremptory summons to attend upon the presences of princes. When a wizened Bedou with a camel stick walked into the surgery at the zoo in Al Ain or found me unerringly in the desert by means of the Empty Quarter version of the bush telegraph, I was expected to drop everything, including an artery of some dying gazelle clamped in forceps or a bottle of artificial plasma dripping slowly into the jugular of an oryx, and go. 'His Excellency must see you at once, *imshi minfadlik*,' the minion would say, spitting into the sand. 'Please come now.'

Ignoring his arrogant stare, I would finish the job in hand, tie off, stitch up, swab clean and then follow him to the land-cruiser waiting nearby with its engine running. It might mean a four-hour drive south and then a ferry boat across to one of the private offshore islands as in the case of Abu Al Abyat, the 25-kilometre-long, completely flat island belonging to Sheik Khalifa, the Crown Prince. This strange place, a barren plain of white sabkha, a mixture of gypsum salt and sand, lies in the clear blue waters of the Gulf, fifty miles south of Abu Dhabi. Its shore is fringed in parts by low, exhausted mangroves but otherwise it is totally void of features. The ground can change quickly from firm going to impassable quicksand within hours, depending upon the subterranean tidal pressure and the temperature. The white sabkha burns in the sun and merges in the near distance on all sides into the shimmering white of the sky. It is a place of mirages and no natural sweet water. How appropriate is its name, Abu Al Abyat – Father of Whiteness.

Yet on this literally white hell live an unknown number of exotic creatures. No-one knows to the nearest five hundred how many there are of wildebeest, antelope, gazelles, zebras or even giraffes. His Highness had populated the island over the years with several thousand rare hoof-stock and had provided water and forage which was taken from the mainland and distributed to hay-racks and troughs across the island by workers employed at his palace and falcon houses, the only buildings on Abu Al Abyat. Once transported to this fiery, inhospitable land, the animals had scarpered into the perpetual heat haze. It was known that many had died – bleached corpses had been found on the sabkha – but not how many survived.

So wild were the animals and so unstalkable because of total absence of cover that one of them had to be in extremis before a Pathan or Pakistani worker could grab it and send for help. When I first visited the island in 1980, it was to examine a Dorcas gazelle found dying of what I diagnosed as septicaemia. Driving cautiously across the white crust of the sabkha, fearful of the invisible bogs that could engulf a vehicle within seconds, I often almost lost my orientation in three dimensions. I was floating in the centre of a white flame – a dream-like and disturbing sensation. Surrounded completely by refracting layers of hot air and travelling over a surface flat as the icing on a cake, the mirages when they came were clear and convincing. A second sun of molten silver would materialise a few yards in front of the vehicle and I would brake hard for fear of falling into its pool of smoking fire. The minaret of the island's palace mosque, a dozen kilometres away, would dance on the tip of the land-cruiser's bonnet, its pierced walls streaming pink and orange flame. And the animals' black silhouettes – the curved horns and beards of the wildebeest, the prickly ears and stamping feet of the zebras and the long necks of the giraffes – appeared as single individuals or as a group amid the rippling silky waves of air. But as soon as I turned and drove towards them, dart gun at the ready, binoculars uncased, they would fade into the whiteness like phantoms. One moment an addax wreathed in vapour sniffed the breeze fifty yards away, the next there was nothing but empty miles of simmering salt and sand.

Our attempts to survey the fauna of Abu Al Abyat were repeatedly thwarted by the mirage. Staking out the food and water points proved useless because the animals were nervous and quick to avoid ambushes. Many of the species are too small to be darted from helicopters. When the Crown Prince recently suggested that all the animals be taken off the island and re-housed in the zoo in Al Ain, I advised caution before Chris, my assistant, promised anything. The Father of Whiteness will not, in my opinion, give up his now well-established children – they are there to stay, protected by Abu Al Abyat's ever-trembling whiteness from further human interference.

About seventy miles to the west of Abu Al Abyat and halfway between Abu Dhabi and Qatar is another island. Where Abu Al Abyat belongs on some strange planet, Sir Bani Yas is at least part of this earth. It has low hills and a little scrub vegetation, and near Sheik Zayed's beach palace there is a tiny airstrip manned by a bored contingent of the UAE air force.

Sheiks are in the habit of presenting grandiose gifts to one another. In the Gulf such presents often take the form of animals that are not infrequently unexpected, unwanted and sometimes downright inconvenient – a handful of male ostriches or a litter of tiger cubs perhaps. Ambassadors visiting the potentates and favour-currying politicos likewise have a tendency to drop in with inappropriate birds and mammals for which the recipients are not prepared and perhaps do not care. That is why every week, out of the blue, consignments of big

85

cats, eagles and the like arrive at the Al Ain zoo. The sheiks are too polite to decline the gifts, but they simply pass them on to the zoo when their visitors leave and then we have the problem of finding quarters, trying to introduce new members into established social groupings, quarantining to prevent the entry of exotic disease and getting vaccination, good nutrition and contraception under way.

It is strange how diplomats manage to lay their hands on priceless endangered species – monkey-eating eagles, Komodo dragons and Japanese falcons – and cart them round the world. But with the universal need to make obeisance at the court of King Oil, those who make animal conservation legislation find no difficulty in breaking it when required. The Arab sheiks of the Gulf are in fact quite selective in their taste in animals, and their zoological likes and dislikes are not what most of their supplicants might surmise. They don't much like eagles, two-humped camels, parrots, toucans, wolves, pigs, leopards, kangaroos, bears or reptiles. If you fancy your chance at getting a contract to supply, say, Lancashire black puddings to the Emirate of Umm al Qaiwan, try winning friends and influencing people by any of the following: deer, gazelles, antelopes, hawks, bustards, Jacob's sheep, ostriches, finches and cheetahs.

In 1981 Sheik Zayed received a gift of ten thousand young pheasants from a nobleman in Dubai. He wasn't familiar with the bird and ordered them to be sent to Sir Bani Yas, that little barren island, where they were housed in large wire-mesh enclosures with shelters made of wood and palm fronds. After some time the Indian labourers who tended the birds noticed signs of sickness developing, and increasing numbers of pheasants began to die each day. The word was passed along the chain of command and quickly reached the ears of His Highness Sheik Zayed himself. 'Send for the English zoo doctor!' he commanded one of his court as he sat sipping sherbet in the pavilion of his beach palace in Abu Dhabi. At once a black Lincoln Continental carrying four Bedou in turbans and white robes with automatic rifles on their laps set out to drive north to the oasis at Al Ain.

When they arrived I was in the surgery, blending a sticky mixture of lanolin and hydrocortisone ointment for a hippo who, dozing too long out of water, had been sunburnt along its back. Chris Furley had gone to the Far East on leave and I was holding the fort – 'Beau Geste' style, I sometimes thought. There was much for me to do, with many animals within the zoo needing constant supervision of medical and surgical conditions. As well as the hospitalised animals in their loosebox 'wards' in the quarantine area – some on fluid drips, some awaiting operations to remove obstructions from their stomachs or amputations of gangrenous toes – there were the daily lists of gazelles, ibex and oryx out in the vast desert enclosures that needed stalking and tranquillising by dart gun in order to discover the cause of their lameness, purulent eyes or lack of appetite. What I could well have done without was the sort of summons borne by four gun-toting Bedou emissaries.

However, one cannot say 'La, la, la', the Arabic 'no', on these occasions. A refusal would not have meant an unsheathing of scimitars or years in a dungeon worthy of Haroun al Rashid – the Gulf Emirates, though still remarkably feudal and un-changed in many ways, tend to mete out ancient Islamic punishments such as stoning, amputation and beheading for only the most serious crimes nowadays – but 'La, la, la' to a great sheik these days could mean visa trouble.

There was no point in going alone to Sir Bani Yas; I would need an interpreter. Luckily Dr Qassan, my accomplice in the failed attempt to reveal to Sheik Jamal the true nature of *radad*, was on site. He agreed to accompany me and, after hurriedly throwing some instruments, sample bottles and drugs into the Bag (which, packed with basic essentials, accompanies me everywhere), we set out together in his car, driving through the desert behind Sheik Zayed's men in their Lincoln.

We swept down the long road between the dunes, probably

one of the most dangerous in the world. Every few yards a mangled car-wreck in the sand and occasional dead camel testifies to the maniacal driving habits of the Emirates. Parallel to the road, camel trains were moving up to Dubai for the next week's races, their young and ragged riders framed against the pink and purple sky of early evening, while outside the bleached tents of small Bedou encampments nestling beneath the nearest dunes, men knelt on scraps of carpet amid their herds of black goats and prostrated themselves towards the setting sun and Mecca. We stopped at a roadside shack to buy 7-Up and dates as darkness fell and then pressed on again for the capital town. At last we arrived at the first of several sentry posts outside the beach palace. Our Bedou escort talked to the guards and we were waved through into the gardens where illuminated fountains sparkled among oleanders and euphorbias while marbled pavilions, pergolas and towers glowed with multi-coloured fairy lights like Blackpool Pier in October.

Dismounting, we went into one of the pavilions, an oblong building with pierced screen walls. Inside, along the centre length of the white alabaster floor, ran a sandpit in which were spiked about twenty cloth- and leather-covered falcon blocks where patient peregrines perched, cocking their heads to survey newcomers with eyes of liquid jet. On the floor around the walls were placed an abundance of cushions and telephones. Bedou sprawled on the cushions conversing quietly in twos and threes, fiddling with their camel sticks or talking on the telephone. A servant moved around with sweet red suleimani tea in tiny transparent cups. 'We must wait here,' said Qassan. 'His Highness will come eventually. Feel free to use the 'phone, David.'

'But . . .'

'Please, do you not have any calls to make – your home, Dr Greenwood, the USA?'

I looked round. Nearly everyone seemed to be on the blower now, one of the perquisites of being in a prince's house. Within the palace of a sheik, guests, minions, visitors and supplicants

88

all submit to a regime of unpredictable and fascinating mediaeval autocracy. Here any man, even the poorest nomad, could bring a petition and, if he were lucky, have it dealt with on the spot by his great lord at one of the daily majlis, or audiences. Feuds could be settled, ownership of camels or disputed betrothals adjudicated. A maker of ornate falcon hoods and jesses, a Palestine Liberation Organisation fund-raiser, the German Ambassador, an Islamic scholar from Al Azhar – all might receive instant, extravagant favour or go away empty-handed with nothing but tea and some free long-distance calls to show for their hours of waiting. Europeans who had converted publicly to Islam would be certain to receive a gift of 60,000 dirhams (about £10,000) or more and purveyors of the latest line in aphrodisiacs were always guaranteed a sale.

Ringing home, I received an updating of the latest happenings in other parts of our far-flung practice from Hanne. 'Andrew's paddling about in the rain in a penguin pool at Cotswold Wildlife Park,' she said, 'while you're among the houris in what sounds like Ali Baba's cave.' Then I settled back onto my cushion and sipped my tea, trying to out-stare the peregrine closest to me.

An hour passed. Then, in a press of soldiers, courtiers, servants, an imam wearing a grey cassock and round red fez, and white-smocked Arab boys with lace skull-caps and camel sticks, there entered a tall and striking figure in a brown robe edged with gold. Aquiline nose, eyes of toasted almond set in a humane face, skin like saddle-leather and glossy black beard – this was Sheik Zayed. He stopped in the pool of light outside the pavilion doorway but didn't come in. We and the others who had been awaiting him moved to join the crowd of followers. Sheik Zayed watched us take up our positions without making any sign of acknowledgement and then set off again through the garden to a white stone palace where lights glowed behind rows of sinuously arched windows and doorways.

Some of the throng seemed to melt away to the garden and only perhaps fifty or sixty of us entered the palace, passing directly into a great banqueting hall glittering with mirrors, chandeliers and gilded wood. When all were seated, troops of servants entered with silver trays of lamb, rice, dates, fresh green peppers and water melon, and dinner began. Brown arms reached out everywhere and wiry fingers tore pieces from the sides of piping hot meat. Sheik Zayed dominated conversation at table and was obviously a talented and witty raconteur. Although I couldn't understand the language I did manage to grasp what he was telling his guests about and Qassan confirmed later that I had indeed got the gist.

His Highness had recently been hunting in Pakistan and while there had stayed in a palace near which stood a mosque whose muezzin wakened the faithful as was the custom at daybreak, when the first light was at last sufficient to distinguish between a black thread and a white, to make their prayers and think about going to work. The problem was that this particular muezzin had a most unpleasant voice. Sheik Zayed imitated the screeching howl of the man as he stood on the balcony of the minaret and cried the ancient invitation, 'Allahu akbar . . .' All the Arab guests roared with laughter at the Sheik's impersonation of the unfortunate caller to prayer, and then began the sort of conversation that one frequently hears among Christians when they discuss the preaching styles or the idiosyncrasies of delivery of their local vicar or non-conformist minister. A Bedou sitting next to me rose to his feet as soon as Sheik Zayed had finished his story and rattled out a description of an even worse muezzin that lived near him. 'Allah oooooohh akbaaaaar!' he screamed. 'Allah oooooohh! The assembled company clapped their hands and chortled in delight.

Now, not to be outdone, each Arab vied with the next to cap the story of the one before by imitating his own nominee for 'minaret monster of the month'. 'Allah akbaaaaaaar! Allah-hoo-ak-ak-ak-baaaar-hoo!' echoed round the room. Every

90

nicety of awful enunciation and unmelodious braying was demonstrated and thoroughly relished by the appreciative listeners. It was a veritable 'knock the local minister' fiesta but done, of course, by men whose faith in and daily observance of the rites of Islam governs their whole lives in a way unique in the Moslem world. It was hilarious, and I joined in the laughter because it really was funny and done in the unspiteful yet knowing way that good Catholics revel in the foibles of their priest or Anglican pillars of the Church bring their rector down to earth.

After the meal, Sheik Zayed lost no time in rising and going to his private bathroom to wash. The rest of us did likewise in a gents' toilet adjoining the banqueting hall, and reminiscent in size and decoration of the one at Waterloo Station. Cleansed from my smearing of lamb, rice and melon, I joined Qassan outside. 'Now you must try to speak to His Highness,' said my companion. 'When he comes out of his bathroom I will approach him.' When the sheik did emerge, Qassan at once walked up to him, bowed and began talking in low tones. Presently he beckoned to me.

'Salaam aleikum,' I said as I shook hands with the great lord. 'Salaam aleikum, Doctor.'

'His Highness wishes you to go to Sir Bani Yas and examine the pheasant birds,' interpreted Qassan. 'Please go and then come back here to report. His Highness will instruct the air force to provide a 'plane.'

It was decreed – and so it happened. A prince of the blood royal, an officer in the Ruler's guard, was at once assigned to us. A limousine was whistled up and we set off without delay. At the airport our escort conducted us into a VIP lounge that was surrounded by unsavoury-looking characters in ill-fitting suits and half a week's growth of beard. Two of them frisked us as we entered and confiscated, without a word, the pen aerosol of undertakers' disinfectant that I carry for emergencies in underdeveloped countries. Inside the lounge we sat drinking Coca-Cola while more unfriendly characters identical to those outside stood over us. Sitting in the armchair next to me was yet another jowly, taciturn man in need of a Gillette. It was Yasser Arafat, and the 'heavies' that littered the place were his minders.

Our prince disappeared and returned half an hour later to say that an aircraft had been prepared for us. We went out and climbed aboard the waiting Learjet. Twenty minutes flight over the Gulf, with the sea shining in full moonlight, and we landed in Sir Bani Yas where the whole of the resident UAE air force detachment turned out to welcome us and help us sort out the pheasant problem. It is not easy, examining ten thousand pheasants in wire pens by the light of Range Rovers' headlamps, but with the help of the Sheik's bird keepers, the airmen and Qassan, I managed to catch a score of them. They were in a parlous state. Many were lame and had swollen joints. Feather-plucking was rife and some birds were almost completely bald over their entire bodies. All were underweight and seemed badly nourished.

'What do you feed the pheasants on?' I aksed the workers.

'The food that is sent from the mainland, Doctor,' came the reply. 'The special bird food.'

I sent for a bag of the special bird food and dug a hand in. I watched the brown flakes sift through my fingers. It was pure bran. 'Nothing else? You give nothing else?' I asked.

'But no, Doctor. We have our instructions.'

I had little doubt that the cause of all the trouble was malnutrition and, giving orders for half a dozen very old birds to be killed, I performed a rudimentary post mortem examination on them in the headlamps' beam. The pitiful carcasses were anaemic and devoid of fat stores. The bones were rubbery and fractured in places. No doubt about it – plain bad feeding was to blame. Bran is a useful poultice for horses and a provider of fibrous bulk in the diets of mammals from humans to donkeys, but by itself it isn't a rich, balanced or valuable food for anything, not even mealworms. Pheasants naturally feed on grain, seeds, shoots and insects; in captivity they must be provided with a pelleted food, similar to that used for poultry, containing balanced amounts of protein, starch, vitamins and so on.

We stayed on the island overnight, sleeping in the Sheik's palace which was infested with heavy, blundering cockchafers that crash-landed into me with monotonous regularity as I lay sweating in the humidity. Early the following morning, after breakfasting on *ful*, a mush of purple beans, raw onions and Arab bread, we flew back to Abu Dhabi to report to Sheik Zayed on my findings. He was no longer at the beach palace but had gone north. The guards were reluctant and evasive when answering Qassan but hinted that we might find him at 'Hadega Gazlan' – the Garden of Gazelles, an estate fifty miles away.

Sheik Zayed was at the garden when we got there, inspecting some of his falcons housed in wooden buildings on the top of a small hill where the wind kept it airy and cool. 'Well, Doctor,' he said after we had waited for him to finish selecting new hoods of lamé and embroidered chamois leather for his pets, fitting them personally over the mewing birds' heads, 'what of these, what do you call them, pheasants?'

'Sir, they are very ill. They are suffering from severe protein deficiency.'

The Sheik threw the veil of his headdress over one shoulder and raised bushy eyebrows as Qassan explained. Then he continued, 'And what medicine do you suggest, Doctor?'

'A change of food, your Highness. Game crumbs, finely chopped meat, lucerne meal, . . .'

'Food? Food? But they receive food. I have sent many tons of food to Sir Bani Yas for them.'

'Yes, you have, sir. But it is bran – not good enough.'

Sheik Zayed gave a loud snort. '*Kalaam faarigh*! Nonsense! Listen, Doctor. The food that you call bran has been good for the other birds I have kept – pigeons for the hawks, chickens and ducks. Are you claiming it is not good enough for these . . . pheasants?'

93

'Yes, I am, sir.'

He glowered at me for a second or two and then clicked his fingers. 'So be it, so be it,' he said. 'If these pheasants are such fussy birds, I lose my patience. Take them to the zoo. I am done with them.'

'But, sir – ten thousand pheasants!'

'To the zoo, Doctor!' The muezzin on the turret of the garden's private mosque began the midday call to prayer. I remember he had a most mellifluous voice. 'I must go to pray now, Doctor. Please clear my island of these troublesome birds.' The Sheik turned on his sandalled heels and walked away towards the mosque, whisking the flies with his camel stick.

More unwanted stock for the zoo: ten thousand pheasants would need a lot of housing and many trips by aircraft and trucks carrying crates to transport them. But the Sheik had spoken and there was no alternative. 'If you hadn't said change the food but simply recommended adding something to cure the disease – medicine, drugs, pheasant pellets, insectivorous food, lucerne or whatever – it would have been OK,' said Qassan as we drove back to Al Ain. 'Medicine is an all-embracing term and he understands that, but you told him that his choice of food had been wrong, so either he or the birds had to lose face. Sheik Zayed never loses face. Now we've got to move the accursed things.'

At the roadside I saw a dead camel that hadn't been there the day before. A black kite sat on its head, neatly shelling out one eye. It was true: I had blown it with Sheik Zayed as surely as I had done with Sheik Jamal thanks to my well-intentioned display of the marvels of the microscope. There is always something new to learn in Arabia.

6 The Egg-Bound Emu

George, the Californian sea-lion at Woburn Abbey, was so named because when young she was thought to be a male. By the time she was bought by Terry Nutkins, my companion on the trip to Macau, her true sex had long been established and she was pregnant. In due course a perfect little female pup was born in the dolphinarium at Woburn, but within hours it quickly became clear that George wasn't interested in suckling her offspring. Terry and I had to make a rapid decision: to struggle for a while, hoping that George would have a change of heart, and give her pituitary gland hormones by dropper into her nose to stimulate let-down of milk; or to attempt artificial rearing.

Sea-lion births in captivity are not very common and successful bottle-feeding of the young can prove difficult, but we'd had encouraging results in recent cases at the Welsh Mountain Zoo and at Ouwehands Zoo in Holland. Buster, a pup born at Chessington Zoo, was at the time being brought up and gaining normal weight on a mixture of blended herring, double cream, cod liver oil and water. We decided to opt for the artificial rearing of George's baby, whom Terry and his wife, Jackie, decided to name Gemini.

As is always the way with sea-lions, things didn't go easily to start with. Terry had to try out many kinds of rubber teat with various sizes of hole before finding one that Gemini seemed happy with. In the first ten days we modified the fishy artificial milk perhaps a dozen times, adjusting the percentages of the constituents and adding milk powder and unsaturated fatty acids. Ordinary milk powders of the sort used for human babies or puppies can prove lethal for seals and sea-lions because of the lactose or milk sugar that they contain; the intestines of sea mammals do not produce the enzymes capable of digesting these chemicals. Terry fed the tiny bundle of short brown fur every hour round the clock and, as soon as Gemini showed symptoms of collywobbles, diarrhoea or loss of appetite, rang me to discuss the next step. Occasionally there were more alarming episodes with colicky pains and sickness; then Terry would jump into his car and bring Gemini down to see me at Lightwater. One summer evening when she was only five days old, we relieved the baby's intestinal cramps with gentle warm enemas administered on the terrace behind my house.

Gradually gemini's system adjusted to the man-made diet. The pup was in good hands because Terry has great empathy with animals and had raised the young of many difficult species including otters. Determined and strong, he was able to handle Gemini when she grew to a size at which I decided to begin early weaning. There would be several benefits, particularly improved condition and more rapid weight-gain if Terry could get the sea-lion on to solid food. Sea-lions don't wean easily; they require weeks and sometimes months of force-feeding before they catch on to the idea of swallowing sprats, mackerel and herring. With jaws far stronger than those of a big dog and a powerful, slippery body, they can be extremely hard to handle. Terry had lost most of three fingers years before, working with Gavin Maxwell's otters, yet he successfully straddled the unco-operative seal-lion five times a day, even when she weighed over sixty pounds, prized open the mouth and stuffed whole fish down the throat. To minimise the chance of Terry being bitten (sea-lion bites can be severe and sometimes lead to a strange and very painful infection called seal finger or blubber finger that used to be common among whalers and sealers in the olden days), I supplied him with a pair of whelping forceps, the instrument used in obstetrical work on bitches. The round grasping ends and long handles could introduce a fish into Gemini's throat and cut the risk to Terry's remaining fingers. But we found the forceps clumsy

96

and insensitive; Terry quickly discarded them and reverted to the riskier digital technique.

As Gemini had been taken from George shortly after birth, she became imprinted on (psychologically bound to) Terry, her foster father. For her Terry was Dad, a bull sea-lion with two legs. Or perhaps Gemini thought herself a rather slithery human being. Certainly as the months passed and the weaning progressed to the point where Gemini would voluntarily accept all fish, it became clear that the sea-lion would feed only in the presence of Terry and, much later, Jackie. If Terry was absent Gemini would not eat a scrap. One, two, three days could pass and Gemini would steadfastly ignore squid, sardines or finest herring proffered by anyone other than Dad – Terry. As soon as the latter returned, however, the animal at once began to eat normally.

This meant that Gemini could never be left for long. Terry and Jackie bought a lovely house on the Isle of Skye, close to the water's edge at Kylerhea with a backdrop of steep mountain slopes. It was a spectacular place abounding with seals, otters, golden eagles, porpoises and pine martens. The young Californian sea-lion slipped easily and naturally into the scenery with a custom-built swimming pool in a converted boat house, rambles along the shore with her master to explore rock pools and the outfalls of streams, and regular runs by car down to Bristol to star in the BBC 'Animal Magic' programme. Gemini grew up in front of the millions of weekly television viewers; they watched her take her first fish, discover her instinctive affinity with water, make acquaintances with a host of other animals from dolphins and dogs to human babies in the form of Terry's daughter and my god-daughter, Jennifer Jane, and even go down to London to make a record with Johnny Morris, Johnny doing the singing and Gemini 'oink-oinking' appropriate sound effects!

Gemini was a healthy, happy sea-lion and, apart from some curious bald patches on her skin which I treated with vitamin H but which probably cleared up on their own account, I didn't have to do any doctoring of the young sea-lion after she was fully weaned. Gemini lived as one of the Nutkins' household and she was never left alone. Always Terry or Jackie were around, although gradually by the time she was two years old she was persuaded to accept fish from other close friends of the family.

As the star of 'Animal Magic', Gemini developed a great following and there were plans for Terry to write her auto-biography. Californian sea-lions are not easy to obtain; they are seldom offered for sale by zoos and breed infrequently in captivity. Their export and import is strictly controlled by tough conservation legislation, particularly on the part of the US Government, and the price of an unacclimatised, un-trained, stranded pup, if one successfully obtains all the necessary permits, may run to around £2,000 excluding transport. Such foundlings, which are the only animals which the Americans allow to be taken at present, are often in poor condition and need a great deal of work and attention before they are in good enough shape to travel. So Gemini must have been worth £20,000 by the time of her second birthday in 1982. 'You really ought to insure her,' I told Terry on several occasions. 'She's becoming as important to your TV career as Roy Rogers' "Trigger". Suppose, just suppose, something happened to her.' Sea-lions are pretty tough creatures; they don't fall ill as easily as dolphins but they can occasionally succumb to the sudden overwhelming infections caused by microbes called Clostridia that are more usually associated with common and important disease epidemics in sheep and which were responsible for the terrible gas-gangrene cases among soldiers in the trenches during the First World War. But whereas a magician who loses a white rabbit or a couple of doves can easily find replacements for his act, and while the 'Flipper' series of television programmes were made using a number of different dolphins in the main part (all bottle-nosed dolphins look alike to laymen), a sea-lion like Gemini was unique. There could never be a substitute.

98

Terry's view was that if anything did happen to Gemini, no cash payment could make up for all that the sea-lion meant to him. With all the care that he lavished upon her, selecting the finest herring and mackerel and supplementing her diet with a comprehensive range of vitamins and minerals, he couldn't, at first, see why she should not attain the ripe old age of twenty or twenty-five. Why, female Californians had even lived for thirty years. For some reason, though, I continued to nag Terry over the question of insuring the quite patently hale and hearty Gemini. Terry eventually agreed to take out a policy on Gemini and I approached the 'Fur, Fin and Feather' consortium of underwriters and brokers at Lloyd's who specialise in covering unusual livestock.

Although many dolphins and most whales are insured by Lloyd's of London, surprisingly few other exotic animals are. Though zoo animal prices are generally rocketing – a king penguin can fetch £3,500, an elephant £10,000 and a rare antelope such as an Arabian oryx £30,000 – insurance is usually only for transport risk when animals are being moved. Premiums can be very high at 20% to 30% for tropical birds, or remarkably low at around 10% for all-risks cover for a killer whale.

Over the years I had often been consulted on problem cases by members of the Lloyd's consortium. Once they had been asked to insure a thousand crocodiles in Bangkok for a total sum of one million dollars; 'Don't do it,' I had advised. First of all, how could one possibly count one thousand crocodiles kept most likely in a muddy pool? And anyway, such a large number of reptiles would be impossible to house and maintain properly and healthily in one place: there was too much chance of disease and what the insurance profession call 'moral hazard' – the possibility of things being fiddled. I again gave a thumbs-down when an underwriter was asked to quote for the insurance of a 'blue lobster' in a North American aquarium for the neatly rounded sum of one million dollars. All lobsters are 'blue' before being cooked and substitution of the crustacean, or indeed perfect murder (invertebrates are easily killed by tampering with their watery environment in ways that would be impossible to detect at post mortem), could have been too readily engineered.

On the other hand, I happily went along with the arrangements drawn up some years ago between Lloyd's and the Cutty Sark whisky company for insuring the life of 'Nessie', the Loch Ness monster, should she be captured alive. Not much chance of substitution in that case, I reckoned!

The underwriters agreed to insure Gemini and, what was more, the Lloyd's Committee let BBC cameras onto the floor of Lloyd's to watch Terry and the sea-lion receive their official policy after I had handed over my certificate of health. Gemini had a riotous day in London. Weighing around seventy-five pounds by now, she wasn't easy for Terry to carry and, when put down, would dash off on exploratory forays in the august surroundings of Lloyd's great hall, barking enthusiastically and playfully snapping at the pin-striped legs of startled city gentlemen doing deals. When we drove round Westminster in a fine Rolls-Royce for linking shots, she leaned out of the open window to make lunges at folk on the pavement, sometimes actually managing to latch hold briefly of a neatly furled umbrella or pigskin briefcase. So long as Terry was around she was happy and, like a faithful and possessive dog, her nips at the uniformed commissionaires, messenger boys and members of the bowler hat brigade who gathered around us during the filming were warning shots in the serious, self-appointed business of protecting her beloved master while he was in the big smoke.

Six months later I was in Antibes, wrestling with Kim's continuing problems, when Terry phoned me. As soon as I heard my friend's voice, I knew that something terrible had happened. He was in Wales with Jackie and the children for a few days holiday. For the first time in the three and a half years of her life, Gemini had been left back at home in Skye without any member of the family in attendance. She was being fed in

100

her spacious boat house by a kind Scotsman who knew her well and was one of the 'strangers' from whom she would accept fish. That morning he had entered the boat house and found Gemini lying dead.

I was as stunned as Terry. Apparently the sea-lion had eaten well and behaved normally on the previous day. 'Do you think it could be poisoning?' asked Terry. 'Something in the fish?'

It was a possibility; what I must do without any delay was an autopsy. 'Go back up to Scotland and meet me at Inverness Airport,' I said. 'I'll get the next plane to London.' Hanne met me when I landed, gave me fresh clothes, a pack of knives, dissecting instruments (the sort that break down and aren't picked up by the security x-rays at airports and cause inconvenient delays or, as often happens with long surgical scissors that Andrew and I use, are actually confiscated), some sample bottles and a quick kiss before I dashed for the Inverness flight. Five hours after leaving Nice Airport I was being ferried across the narrow straits separating the mainland from the Isle of Skye by a grim-faced Terry.

We walked up the road to his house and went straight to the boat house. Inside Gemini lay as if she were peacefully sleeping. There was a small pool of vomit by her head. Together we carried her outside to a place behind the house on a grassy slope at the foot of the hillside. The evening light was fading fast and we had to work with the aid of storm lanterns. It must have been hard for Terry to watch, hold forceps and seal sample bottles as I began to cut into the body of his devoted friend. The autopsy was straightforward. Only one thing could I find that was in any way abnormal: the entire liver was swollen, spongy and an unusual coppery colour. Gemini had died from acute hepatitis. The laboratory tests were later to show that this was indeed the cause of death – an overwhelming destruction of liver cells by virus particles.

Where had the virus come from? What kind of virus was it? These questions have not yet been answered. Viruses are mysterious entities, in some ways behaving as living things and

101

in other ways, displaying the properties of inanimate chemical molecules. Perhaps Gemini's virus had come from some other animal in the neighbourhood – an otter, a mouse or a fish. We just don't know enough about the life history of viruses, particularly those which may affect marine mammals. Human influenza viruses are thought sometimes to 'hide' in pigs between epidemics. Every year new viruses are found emerging from the jungles of Africa and South America. Mutations are constantly occurring and some viruses can lie dormant in certain species for years. Laboratory work on viruses, particularly of the sort that we found in Gemini, is difficult; there aren't sea-lions around to be used as laboratory guinea-pigs and tissue culture lines of sea-lions cells simply don't exist in the United Kingdom. Perhaps I will never know the exact nature of Gemini's virus, and I sometimes wonder if it was a coincidence that she died on the first occasion of being separated from Terry and Jackie or whether a degree of psychological stress lowered her physical resistance.

Gemini was buried on Skye and with her ended one of the most interesting and successful human/wild animal relationships that I have come across. With her passing Terry and Jackie lost more than a friend; their beautiful home on Skye would never be the same again and they began making plans to move back down to England.

Midwife to monkeys, meerkats, mongooses and mountain lions I have been in my time. I have held the hand, or hoof, or paw, of thousands of exotic mothers-to-be, given 'twilight sleep' gas to orang-utans with breech presentations, been shoulder-deep with both arms in the birth canal of a giraffe that was having difficulties with an oversized calf and done Caesarean operations on complicated cases in zebras, tigers, tapirs and gazelles in the blazing midday heat of the desert to the bitter 3 am cold of a winter's night in Scandinavia. In twenty-five years of zoo practice I had seen live calves with six legs, apes with 'hole in the heart' blue babies, leopard cubs

102

without anuses and zebra foals that needed supports for broken necks, but I have never been obstetrician to a bird bigger than a budgerigar. Egg-bound budgies are ten-a-penny. Thank goodness, I used to think, that bigger birds like ostriches, cassowaries and emus – the heavy mob among our feathered friends, with outsize tempers and mayhem-mindedness to match their size – seem always to deliver their young parcelled up in eggs without benefit of veterinarian.

So it was until I met Clara, the Chessington emu. All flightless birds except penguins are well compensated for their lack of wings by the possession of powerful legs and feet and mean beaks with which they vent their accustomed choler on curators, chance trespassers into their territory, admirers of their womenfolk, young or eggs and, naturally, veterinary surgeons. Should they fancy it, they can bite, disembowel, belabour or simply stomp on you. This latter, I knew from bitter experience, gives them the added pleasure of publicly humiliating the miserable human who is the object of their blitzkrieg. You lie with your face pressed into the soil while an overgrown turkey with feet the size of shovels does an accurate ornithological impression of a drunken disco-dancing dope fiend with painful piles up and down your spine. In front of the public, erstwhile admiring students or girl friends who came along to see 'what wonderful things you do for the animals', you lose face – if nothing else!

Despite their unpredictable aggressiveness and wickedly strong legs, however, flightless birds are weak in the head and in the heart. Rather stupid creatures, they also have hearts which can flake out with alarming suddenness. Putting a sack on the head of, say, an ostrich in the same way that one tries to calm a horse may stop its accurate kicking and lunging but may also induce a fatal cardiac arrest. My preferred method of coming to grips with these ratites, as flightless birds are called, is to dash in quick with two or three men and seize the beast before its tiny brain has had time to plot murder. Standing as close as possible to the legs, with arms round base of neck, body and meaty thighs, we are safe from attack and have the bird in custody. But make sure everyone keeps their hands off the bird's windpipe because an accidentally throttled ostrich or emu is valueless – the market in feather boas and Kentucky fried cassowary is rock bottom! Live, however, such animals fetch several hundred pounds each.

Now Clara of Chessington was and is an unusual emu with some of the characteristics of the dummy bird used by ventriloquist Rod Hull. The aforementioned 'snatch squad' technique of catching works as well on her as on any other emu. Her difference is that once grabbed, she refuses to call it a day and submit. She continues instead to use her strong beak not for biting or stabbing (it isn't suitable for that) but to pluck. Once restrained in the nether regions, Clara systematically begins to wrench at and pull off bits of her captors' clothing. She does it precisely, takes a good hold and rips. Either the fabric merely tears and affords a better approach for the next pluck, or an area of cloth is completely removed and discarded. She is fast, methodical and underterrable.

Clara was destined to become my first ratite obstetric patient. An emu egg resembles a large avocado pear in size and colour; though not as big as the egg of an ostrich, one made into an omelette would be enough for about six people. Generally between nine and thirteen eggs are laid by the emu hen who then (emu for women's lib!) lets the cock do all the incubating. Why, after successfully laying eleven good eggs, Clara should balk at the twelfth and final one I don't know. But on one summer's day in 1982 that is just what she did. Mick, the senior bird keeper and an old Belle Vue hand, was quick to spot her straining away fruitlessly. After several hours with no signs of progress and the eventual discharge of a small quantity of dark liquid, he notified the curator, Lionel, who in turn phoned me.

'Where are you off to?' asked Hanne as I checked the Bag.

'Chessington, to whelp an emu.'

'What?'

'Unbunging an overgrown Australian chicken!' I smiled at

104

her puzzled expression as I went out of the back door – but Clara was going to wipe that smile off my face in no time at all.

An hour later, with buckets of hot water and disinfectant nearby, Lionel, Mick and I stood ready to mug Clara. I had seen her give a few strong pushes and something was definitely stuck in her works, although not a glimpse of eggshell was visible.

'OK. Everybody ready? GO!' Lionel gave the word and we dashed hell-for-leather through the gate of the emu pen and surrounded the surprised bird. Mick took the front position with one arm hugging her chest and the other in front of her collarbone. Lionel was fully occupied further back, clinging on to the emu's muscular thighs like grim death. For a moment Clara acted nonplussed. Then she sank to the ground, taking her captors with her. Lionel and Mick knelt beside her on the damp earth but didn't relax their holds. I would now have to do my obstetrical investigation at grass roots level rather than the easy-on-my-back height of a standing emu.

I scrubbed my hands and forearms with mercury soap, lubricated them with obstetric jelly and lay on the ground behind Clara's rear end. Then the plucking began. True to form, Clara began to go for bits of our apparel like the first granny in at a jumble sale. Swivelling her head through almost 360 degrees and snaking her long neck down, she zoomed in with her iron-hard black beak. Z-i-i-i-k! Off came half of Lionel's collar. Pop, pop! Two buttons gone from Mick's shirt. I felt a blow between my shoulder blades and cool air on my back as Clara tossed a handkerchief-size scrap of my shirt into the air. There was a ripple of applause and some laughter from the distance – we had an audience of visitors.

Exploring the cloaca of the big bird, I came into contact with the hard, rather dry shell of an egg about a hand's length in. It was jammed tight.

'A-a-a-wk!' Mick yelled in agony. Clara had espied a fashionable gold earring the keeper sported in his right earlobe and latched on to it. 'A-a-a-wk! A-a-a-wk!' Mick was making a painfully accurate impersonation of a tortured parrot. Clara gave the triumphant hollow boom so typical of emus, detached the bauble from the bleeding ear and swallowed it.

Stoically, Lionel and Mick held on. I was in a curious and vulnerable position and had no desire to be left alone with one arm up the fundament of an irate, unrestrained emu. With a hiss, more of my shirt now disappeared. Boom, boom! went Clara. Oh bloody hell – now she was down to Lionel's string vest! She began deftly to enlarge the holes in the latter, changed her mind and returned to Mick. With one appallingly accurate pluck she unzipped his fly. Thank God he was kneeling down. Peck, peck, boom, boom – the keeper's trousers slowly began to slide. The crowd of visitors at the other side of the fence was swelling. Their appreciation of the free show which fitted in neatly between the feeding time for the sea-lions and the first circus performance was heart-warming – for Clara.

Try as I might, I couldn't get anywhere with the egg. I could touch one smooth end of the ovoid and even get a finger an inch or so along the sides, but there was no way of pulling it. The lubricating jelly was dissipating rapidly. I put my other hand under her pelvis and pressed inwards. Perhaps I could squeeze the egg out. Whisk! My collar was rent asunder. The egg stubbornly stayed put.

'Are you nearly there, Doc?' groaned Mick through gritted teeth. I wasn't. I didn't want to break the thing or risk drilling a hole in it to get a purchase. It would just have to slide out. Give me an antelope calf any time, I thought miserably. At least it presents the possibility of between one and four legs, two eyes and a tail to wrestle with.

The obstetric jelly was not giving enough lubrication. What I needed was something greasy. 'Hold on, lads' I said, pulling out. 'I'll be back in a moment.' I left them embracing Clara and ran to the little fish-and-chip bar that stands near the bird garden. 'A paper cup full of cold cooking oil, please,' I said as I went in, pushing my way up to the counter.

The youth shovelling chips into a carton gave me a baleful

glare. 'We don't sell oil separate, mate, and can't you see the queue?'

'I'm the vet here. Give me the oil *now*, please! I'll explain later.' I could hardly risk putting paying customers off their victuals by giving them the idea that pommes frites à la Chessington Zoo are fried in fat that may have been up an emu's bottom!

Grudgingly and with deep suspicion, the boy thereupon provided the cup of oil and, feeling rather like a foolish virgin, I dashed back to Clara, Mick and Lionel. The chip-oil proved a great improvement on the specially formulated obstetric jelly that otherwise seems to work well on great ladies and ungrateful gophers with labour hold-ups. But still the bottle-green egg didn't yield an inch. I sweated away with my nose in the plumage of Clara's rump. Impasse. No egg and chip-oil. There was no substitute for a handle on the egg – but I find that nature doesn't tend to design things with bumbling veterinarians in mind.

Mick had just been partially debagged. His knees on the ground inhibited further trouserial descent but he was valiantly flying the flag – his Union Jack Y-fronts were glowing patriotically in front of the admiring visitors. Clara stared at the Y-fronts with an eye to striking the colours.

A handle. I needed a handle. 'Hold on a minute, lads, I won't be long.'

'Oh no, not again,' my two assistants protested in unison. 'We can't hold on much longer.'

I extracted my now oily arm once more and ran off again into the zoo. Past the fish-and-chip bar, round the polar bears, the mara pen and the flamingo pool. I puffed into the maintenance department. Robin, the clerk of works, was inspecting a batch of newly constructed transport boxes with his men. 'Quick! I need a plunger,' I gasped.

'A what?' He stared at my dishevelled state, shirt in tatters, arms dripping with oil and flustered, sweating face.

'A plunger for unblocking drains. Smallest size'

'You've not clogged up the sink in the post mortem room with cotton wool and unmentionable bits of dead animals again, have you?'

'No. Quick.' I was thinking of Mick, possibly even now totally denuded by Clara. 'I'm trying to unblock an emu.'

I thought the maintenance gang would all expire of apoplexy. When the guffawing subsided and they realised that I was in a far from laughing mood, Robin darted into the plumbing section and quickly came back with a selection of sticks with rubber cups on their ends, simple devices for clearing obstructions in sink drains and the like. I picked the smallest and dashed back to Clara's paddock. The two men and a bird were still locked in the same picturesque tableau, Lionel now naked to the waist and Mick with his gory ear and patriotic underwear looking like a National Front supporter frozen in the act of duffing up a Trot. Clara, however, was the one patiently carrying on with the duffing up. Snip, snap, boom, boom! Her beak had lost none of its punch.

I washed myself once more and then disinfected the plunger as well as I could in povidone. Greasing my hands with the chip-oil, I then carefully introduced the drain-clearer into the emu's cloaca. Guiding it with my fingertips, I positioned the rubber cup against the surface of the egg and gave a little push on the wooden handle. There was a rude noise from inside Clara as the suction took effect. I gently tugged the plunger; it had latched firmly on to the egg. Very slowly, with one hand easing the shell along the delicate membrane of the cloacal canal and the other pulling the stick, I began to move the egg backwards. Millimetre by millimetre it slipped towards me and then I saw the first glint of bottle-green. Rotating the egg to ease its passage, I continued the steady traction. With a satisfying 'thunk' it finally popped out, followed by a noisome mixture of chip-oil, blood and mucus. 'Got it!' I sighed, and reached for syringes to administer a protective injection of sulphur drug.

It was a weary and tattered trio who trudged back to Lionel's office bearing the cause of all our trouble. To look at, it was identical to any other emu egg, neither bigger nor rougher nor more irregular in shape than the next. The zoo paid for a replacement earring for Mick and for three shirts and a string vest. The egg, after careful incubation in the bird house, turned out to be addled and exploded obscenely one morning about a month later while Mick was carefully turning it. The zoo bought yet another shirt for Mick.

The big Indian buffalo at Madrid had developed a huge tumour in a most unusual place – right on the pendulous tip of its brisket. As big as a melon with a neck as thick as my arm, the growth rubbed against the front legs and became red, raw and very ugly. It would have to be removed surgically. Indian buffaloes, very large animals with the longest horns grown by any creature (up to thirteen feet, tip-to-tip), are not as aggressive as African Cape Buffaloes or the small Anoas of the Celebes and Philippines, but they can be dangerous when approached by strangers. I discussed the operation with Liliana and Antonio-Luis, who are undoubtedly the hardest-working and most dedicated zoo veterinarians in Europe. If I have to work with anyone, I prefer it to be with them.

There was no chance of palpating the tumour and then perhaps taking it off under local anaesthetic, as one might do with a domestic cow. We would have to use a cocktail of two anaesthetics after the animal had been denied food and water for twenty-four hours; the trouble with ruminating animals and particularly members of the cattle family is that they tend to regurgitate stomach contents when unconscious. This stuff unfortunately comes back up the throat and out of the nose rather than through the mouth and can therefore easily find its way down into the lungs to cause fatal inhalation pneumonia. With the help of a day's 'starvation' I should be able to operate without much risk. Technically the tumour's size and position presented no difficulties: cut round the neck of the growth in healthy tissue, deal with a few blood vessels and stitch everything up.

It didn't take long for Antonio-Luis, a dab hand with a blowpipe, to dart the buffalo. So light and silent are the blowpipe's darts that the big black fellow treated my friend's injection as if it were no more than a mosquito bite and merely tossed his head a few times. Ten minutes elapsed before the buffalo sank to his knees and then rolled over, eyes closed. As soon as he was unconscious, the three of us entered the pen in which he lay and began the preliminaries. While Liliana gave antibiotics and anti-stress shots, Antonio-Luis checked his heart and lungs with a stethoscope and arranged his legs in a comfortable position, and I knelt on the ground to examine the big tumour in detail. It looked like a benign fibroma, and the neck was too thick for it to be twisted off in the way Mr Herriot & Co. can deal with so-called 'angleberry' warts of the belly and udder in dairy cattle. Next Liliana washed the thing in povidone and painted on skin disinfectant while I arranged the trays of sterile instruments and scrubbed my hands in a bucket of warm water and povidone.

'David – look!' Antonio-Luis called sharply as I finished my preparation.

I looked round. The buffalo had stopped breathing! I fell to my knees and put my stethoscope to his chest. The heart was still beating, but very slowly.

'*Muerto* – dead,' murmured Antonio-Luis, who had lightly touched an eyeball with a finger. There was no reflex closing of the eyelids, merely a glassy stare.

'*Respiracion artificiel!*' I barked. 'You give twenty cc's of doxapram and five of M285 into the jugular, Liliana, while I pump the chest.' My friend's syringe with the antidote had been filled even before we began giving the anaesthetic, and she had another containing the powerful drug that can kick the respiratory control centre in the brain into action. Such precautions weren't just in case something like this happened to the animal; they were also essential life-savers in case one of us humans inadvertently got the tiniest amount of anaesthetic – through a scratch with a needle or a droplet in an eye or on the lips – into our system. The anaesthetic acts so quickly and kills so easily in primates (including man) that an accident case would need instant, on-the-spot attention; ambulances, doctors, hospitals would all be far too late.

You can't give the 'kiss of life' to anything much bigger than a gorilla, and standard human first-aid techniques of artificial respiration don't apply to buffaloes. I jumped onto the motionless animal's chest and reached for the top of some iron fencing above my head. With both hands holding the fencing, I danced up and down on the mighty rib cage like a jack-in-a-box, first stamping down with all my weight to compress the lungs at least partly, then lifting myself up to allow them to expand and suck in the vital air.

Suddenly Antonio-Luis, crouching at the beast's head, taking the pulse and watching for any return of reflexes, groaned. '*Mira*, David! Look what is happening here.' A river of olive-green soup was flowing out of the buffalo's nostril. Despite the day without food and water, it had retained enough stomach fluid to regurgitate.

'That's finished it,' murmured Liliana, who had completed her injections. 'No matter what happens, it will drown itself.'

The buffalo blinked an eyelid. I stopped my Cossack dance on his chest and swung awkwardly from the fence, watching intently. There: the buffalo breathed in a weak lungful and then softly exhaled. It coughed once. It was still alive! If not too much stomach contents had gone down into the lung, I could prevent the pneumonia before it began by giving steroids and a broad-spectrum antibiotic. The only trouble was that now, with the anaesthetic antidote in his system, he should soon be back to consciousness, and with the tumour still untouched. 'At least he's not dead yet,' I said, returning to terra firma. 'Give a big dose of oxytetracycline and some flumethasone. I'm going to have a crack at getting that tumour off in two minutes flat.'

Two minutes was perhaps the most I could expect. No time for fancy surgery but then this shouldn't be a tricky business. No major blood vessels, nerves or organs in the flap of fatty skin that is the brisket. Two great incisions with the scalpel should have the thing off at its base. A bit of bleeding wouldn't trouble such a big creature. No time to tie off any big vessels, but there shouldn't be any. Bang a handful of fibrin foam into the hole and close the wound with two or three giant mattress sutures of braided nylon. All that, I reckoned, could be done in around one hundred seconds.

I reached for a scalpel and bent over the tumour. Yes, two long cuts – the blade would run through that tissue like butter – should do it. But instead of pressing the knife point into the skin and sweeping it swiftly from left to right for six inches, something made me hesitate. Not a six-inch sabre cut, a little voice in my head said, you've still enough seconds to spare. Do it two inches at a time. So I cut the two inches – and at once found myself in big trouble. I had encountered a blood vessel as wide as my finger. What was more, my scalpel blade sliced into it and several other veins which didn't seem to realise they had no anatomical right to be there! Blood was everywhere. With the buffalo beginning to flick its ears and breathe strongly, I was faced with the need to control my hand-made massive haemorrhage.

Feverishly I began to clamp vessels with forceps and tie them off with catgut. I must stop the bleeding and close the hole. All idea of removing the tumour went to the wind. Clamp, tie off, suture was all I could think about. Clamp, tie off, suture. The buffalo was pawing with its massive hooves. Within moments it would be on its feet and once again perfectly able to charge and to wield those enormous horns. The stream of arterial blood slackened as my fingers popped in and out of the wound like bees bringing pollen to the hive. 'Careful, *cuidado!*' yelled Antonio-Luis. 'It's getting up!'

I had two more vessels to tie and one big mattress suture to insert. The buffalo gave a grunt and with a great heave rose to its feet, forceps dangling like silver jewels from its brisket. 'Clear out all the gear except what I'm using,' I said, and knelt in the straw beneath the animal's legs as it stood puffing and collecting its thoughts. 'Please stay like this just a half-minute more,' I prayed silently. I forgot, blocked out, where I was – directly under a ton of wild beef. For me only the trickle of blood, the gut, the nylon and the needle existed in the whole universe. One more stitch. Surely the buffalo wouldn't drop on me, wouldn't back off and scoop me up on those dark horns; some of the drugs in the anaesthetic cocktail, the non-reversible ones, must be, please God, still be-fuddling his brain a teeny weeny bit. 'Good boy. Cush-cush, cush-cush.' I whispered the comfortable words that Lancashire farmers intone as they move among their cows. 'Cush-cush. Cush-cush.' 'There, there' in cow-talk. Anything to keep the seconds passing without the animal changing its position.

Finished! With my fingers sticking together with dried blood, I tied the final knot and then slid away from the buffalo, pulling my instrument tray behind me and without cleaning up the stitch line. As I got to my feet when I was a couple of yards from him, he made an imprecise lunge with a horn and stamped a forefoot. The tumour hung obscenely from his brisket as he turned and walked slowly to the fence to look at the other buffaloes gathered outside, fascinated spectators during the whole of the proceedings.

'Do you think he'll make it?' asked Liliana.

'Probably. I don't think he inhaled too much fluid. Your shots should cope with it.'

'What do we do now?'

'Try again in a few weeks' time after two days without food and one day without water.'

Liliana nodded but looked doubtful. 'But aren't these species always unpredictable under anaesthetic? And might not this one be an oddball anyway? We could get total respiratory collapse next time.'

'Maybe. And I know the animal isn't worth much money. But the tumour can't be ignored. It must come off. If we lose our nerve because of screw-ups like this, we'll gradually start going back to the old days, the old excuses: if in doubt do nothing; leave well alone; take the easy way out; let Nature take its course; suggest to the director it would be cheaper to buy another one. Zoo veterinary surgery depends on us not losing our balls, to put it bluntly.'

Liliana smiled broadly. 'You're right, David. Come on, let's go for a wash and then a San Miguel.'

'Or two,' I replied.

Motherhood had mellowed Shao-Shao, the panda. Her previously unpredictable and sometimes cantankerous attitude towards her keepers and veterinarians was replaced by something akin to geniality. She was proud of her fast-growing cub and seemed delighted to let me take a look at it at quite close quarters. Her milk must have been a rich brew, for the infant was obviously putting on weight far more rapidly than most mammalian young. I would have dearly liked a sample of panda milk for analysis as we have no idea of its make-up, but that was out of the question.

Only once during its first few months did the baby give cause for alarm. In late December 1982 it suddenly missed three of its usual suckling periods. Antonio-Luis phoned me and asked me to be prepared to take the next flight out. I booked a seat on the plane and then the phone rang again. The baby had suddenly started to suckle once more and with gusto. Gladly I cancelled my reservation.

At the beginning of 1983 the baby, now looking like a baby panda rather than a rather curious piglet, was named Chu-Lin by the zoo and we discussed the first vaccination for the youngster. I decided to give the initial injection against panleucopenia (a common disease of domestic cats) when the baby was four and a half months old and then give a special dead distemper vaccine which had been sent to me by the National Zoo in Washington around four weeks later. 19 January 1983, the day after my unsuccessful attempt to take off the buffalo's tumour, was a great day for me: I was going to handle, weigh and then inject my first real live giant panda cub.

Shao-Shao by this time was quite happy to leave the cub alone in her den and go outside to eat her beloved strawberry-flavoured Complan. While she was thus engaged, the plan was for me to go in with a keeper and at last take hold of the precious little black and white bundle. Scrubbed up and wearing a sterile surgical gown and plastic overshoes, I walked through a disinfectant bath and entered Shao-Shao's den. Chu-Lin was rolling unconcernedly about in the thick bedding of wood wool. The keeper picked up the cub and handed it to me. A magical moment!

Chu-Lin really was everything one imagines a baby panda to be. He felt right – cuddly, soft and warm – and he lay in my arms without any of the irritability or impatience of a bear cub of the same age. He didn't smell like a bear cub. His fur was smooth and clean and his eyes – oh, his eyes! They didn't roam like a bear cub's but gazed steadily into mine like those of a human infant. They were dark, shining, clear eyes, totally different from those of any other young animal I have ever seen, and they were tranquil and benign. I lifted one of the upper lips. Chu-Lin didn't complain, and I saw that the gums were a healthy salmon-pink. I pulled down an eyelid – the conjunctiva were clean and well-coloured. The distinctive markings of the baby panda were now fully developed except for the damp little nose which was still pink in parts.

There is a quaint legend among the inhabitants of the mountains of Central China which explains how the panda's black and white livery is supposed to have originated. Once long ago, so they say, pandas were completely white. A young girl befriended the animals and one day saved the life of a baby panda which was being attacked by a leopard, but in doing so she was mortally wounded. When she died the giant pandas attended her funeral wearing black on their shoulders, arms and legs, the traditional Chinese signs of mourning. Moved to tears, the pandas wiped their eyes with their paws and turned them black. Then they held their heads in their paws, blackening their noses and ears. They have borne the marks of grief ever since that day.

How proud I was to be holding this rarest of animals. I had handled snow leopards, gorillas, dolphins, walruses, gazelles and a thousand other species over a quarter of a century but nothing had moved me as much as this. Using a pair of bathroom scales, I tried to weigh Chu-Lin but he wouldn't stay on the weighing platform long enough for us to get a reading. So I took his weight by difference, first weighing myself and then Chu-Lin and me together and subtracting one figure from the other. Eleven kilos! In four and a half months the baby had gone from one hundred grams to eleven kilos, an increase of eleven thousand percent.

Now I had to give the first injection in Chu-Lin's life. I had loaded a syringe with a specially tested and sterilised dead vaccine (the live vaccines might well be safe for cats but I wasn't taking any chances that they might behave differently in a giant panda) and, holding Chu-Lin's scruff like that of a cat, I poked in the needle and pressed the plunger. The baby panda let out one single lusty yell and then seemed to forget all about the prick. When I put him down onto the floor, the baby hurried off to play with a plastic ball. Leaving the keeper to keep Chu-Lin amused for a while I slipped out, elated. As far as I was concerned, I had just reached the peak of my career as a zoo vet.

7 Live With Animals

The man in the pub always says the same thing: 'My lad wants to be a vet. Daft about animals, he is.' The lady in the queue at the post office seems invariably to have a daughter who wants to be a vet but couldn't possibly bear seeing an animal in pain. I've said it before: veterinary medicine isn't all Herriotism, and wild animal medicine is worlds away from *All Creatures Great and Small*. I often reflect on my work – what I am doing and why. The ethical and philosophical aspects of keeping wild animals in captivity are complex and subtle. Am I the equivalent of a prison doctor? Should not all wild animals be free?

There are no simple answers to the many questions raised by the interaction of man and animals on this planet. Nothing is black and white. The anti-vivisectionists and the animal liberationists can no more claim infallibility than the aficionados of the *corrida* or the hunting, shooting, fishing brigade. Britain in 1982 still teems with animal life and one of the least numerous species, the not-so-naked ape with the bowler hat and Union Jack waistcoat, continues to bask in the reputation of being the world's foremost animal-lover. Every year we British contribute more to the RSPCA than to the NSPCC, purchase £250 million worth of tinned pet food and provide the latest in medical attention for 100,000 new cases of heart disease in dogs and cats that succumb to the same spin-offs of affluence, over-eating and under-exercise that afflict their primate owners.

In this country where the most popular sport is not football, but fishing, where you can provide your pooch with a luxury animal hotel for his holidays, get him blood from a canine blood transfusion service if he poisons himself by eating the stuff we lay down to kill rats and mice and at the end inter him with all due pomp and circumstance in a pets' cemetery, where the Labour Party and SDP have declared their intention of banning animals in circuses should they gain office and where guerillas of the Animal Liberation Front give interviews, suitably masked, to television reporters, is it not true that we are as we so often claim *the* nation of animal lovers? Love me, love my dog – cat, budgie, race-horse, pheasant and all the rest? It quickly becomes apparent, if you consider the protestations and love for animals that ninety-nine per cent of homo sapiens make, that some of us interpret 'love' in one way while others mean something rather different. Behind it all, if we bother to think about it, our attitudes are based on a bewildering muddle of illogicality, hypocrisy, sloppy thinking and ignorance.

Although we can obviously like some animals for being pretty, cuddly or even downright comical, and we can be fascinated scientifically by the wonders of the animal kingdom, it is in the area of ethics and morality concerning our fellow creatures that we are most at sea. I suppose the basic problem we 'Christian' British face is the unmistakable fact that on the one hand the Church has no official theological view of animals and on the other hand the science of evolution does not, in my view, permit us to maintain ideas of any special unique divide either in zoological or ethical terms between man and other species situated elsewhere on the ever-growing tree of evolution.

Logically, however life began on this planet, all the evidence of biological evolution from that point onwards shows us to be a sort of ape, successful in our own terms and in the twinkling of an eye that is our own time. But we are no more 'special' or 'unique' than, say, trilobites were in their age or Tyrannosaurus Rex was in its. In an evolutionary sense there is no doubt that monkeys and mice and beyond that Tyrannosaurus and trilobites, right back to the first living organisms in the primeval ooze, are relatives, some close and some more distant. So what attitude do we, should we take towards our 'relatives'? Is it anything more than a concern of self-interest? Has it a moral basis? Did St Francis of Assisi with his 'Brother Ass' and 'Sister Dove' put his finger on something of profound importance to Christian thinking that is infinitely more significant than the comfortable, cosy, allegorical way, perhaps with echoes of the old pantheistic approach to Nature, that they are usually interpreted?

Although other religions such as Buddhism and Hinduism, particularly where there is a belief in re-incarnation, adopt a different attitude towards 'lower' creatures, Christianity is in essence targeted towards one species and one species only. Despite references in the Bible to a whole variety of livestock from snakes to whales to marmots, they play only the smallest incidental walk-on parts. Christianity claims uniqueness for homo sapiens, based on his possession of an extra bit of functional anatomy, the soul.

The Christian attitude to animals, or at least what there is of it in formal terms, has changed only to an extent since it began to follow reluctantly the coat-tails of post-Darwinian science. Historically, the zoological approach of the Church was only a mirror of its times. In the earliest days it was thought that beasts possessed some sort of soul. The great St Thomas Aquinas stated that the souls of animals were not created by God but were 'derived with their bodies from their parents by natural generation' and therefore perished when the body perished. The Christian philosopher, Descartes, denied even so much and claimed animals to be 'mere machines'. The Church has often not been clear even as to what animals are. In mediaeval times the unborn foetuses of rabbits were pronounced not to be meat and therefore suitable food for fast days. Not all that long ago the Church in South America said the same thing about capybaras, the largest member of the rodent family, on the grounds that they live in marshy land that frequently floods and so might conveniently be classified as fish. On the one hand nowadays we have the fundamentalist anti-evolutionists and their recent re-run of the famous 'monkey' trial in the USA, and on the other the clerics who fudge theology with their Animals Day services.

Modern scholastic theology's view of animals is probably that described in my old copy of the *Catholic Dictionary*: 'The brutes are made for man, who has the same right over them which he has over plants and stones.' Brutality is wrong because 'we are apt to become callous, even to human sufferings, and we do wrong to expose ourselves to such a danger, unless on the weighty grounds of a higher benevolence.' In other words, cruelty to animals would be okay if you could be sure that it didn't make you more unfeeling towards your own species. Human beings are special.

The relationship between man and animals has probably always been an uneasy one. Did primitive man ever live in harmony with other species in some ancient ecological paradise? Certainly it is curious how nowadays the only species which is generally regarded as beyond the pale is man. See any mixed group of animals on, say, an African savannah: antelope, zebra, giraffe, elephants and birds move among one another, and even predators, if they obey the rules of time and territory, are accepted. Enter a human being and the atmosphere changes. Domestication of animals, which in the case of the dog probably began as a result of animals being attracted to man's waste deposits, proceeded through symbiosis to exploitation to slavery and sometimes on to even more extreme usage. The definition of exploitation and slavery, the grey areas between one sort of animal/human interaction and another, and the rights and wrongs of them, are what the debate is all about.

If the Garden of Eden relationship between man and other creatures ever existed it has certainly been lost now. Conservation aims in a fragmentary way to move in that direction, particularly where habitat protection can be effective. But even in sanctuaries for, say, gorillas or tigers, man cannot usually be included as part of the ecological balance as one of the indigenous fauna. Modern homo sapiens is essentially a domesticated animal, an artificial product that can exist only in an artificial environment. He can no more be balanced in the ecology of most parts of the earth than dachshunds or English bulldogs could be expected to survive as dogs in the wild.

Symbiosis? Mutual benefit, it seems to me, applies only to some of the most simple animals: bees, for example, although even here we are sometimes guilty of genocide with our chemical sprays and modern garden practices. Exploitation? Certainly. Although we often like to retain the use of the word 'exploitation' for things like broiler beef and battery hens, isn't all animal/man interaction to some extent exploitation, if not indeed true slavery? We control the births, growth and death of a wide number of species. We change their shapes and sizes by artificial selection to suit our tastes – both gastronomic, as in pig-breeding, and aesthetic, as in the creation of fancy breeds. We even mutilate animals for reasons of art as in tail-docking, to promote a certain type of growth as with castration, or to exert control as in ringing bulls. We eat animals, crop them alive, dress them and make them do physical work. We use them as proxies in scientific experiments, as entertainers and as weapons. As St Thomas Aquinas said, 'They have no free will.' Is not some of this a form of slavery; can we not compare the gladiator to the Grand National runner?

We are, of course, rather selective in our likes and dislikes of animals. There is no logic to it. There are 'good' animals like dogs, cats, birds and bunny rabbits and there are 'bad' animals like rats, spiders and centipedes. How we treat animals seems to me to depend on who they are. Even among the bigger creatures we are selective in our attitude. Logic yields to sentimentality and irrationality. Cattle in a slaughter house are shot between the eyes with a captive-bolt pistol. What dog owner would permit a veterinary surgeon to euthanase their pet in the same way? Rats are 'pests', so we give them chemical baits which cause them to haemorrhage painfully, if evidence from accidental dog-poisoning cases is anything to go by, into their joints and body spaces. And what about farm animals in intensive systems? Or the parrot usually alone in a small cage? Or budgerigars or alsatian dogs so commonly kept in council flats? Can we criticise zoos and circuses, let alone safari parks, when such confinement exists?

Apart from the 'good' and the 'bad' animals, it seems to me that there is also another group of 'super' animals, like whales and pandas. Here our selective attitude of mind seems to reach the dizziest heights. The whale nowadays appears to occupy a quasi-mystical place in many people's thinking. Is it not curious that a mammal that few folk have ever seen in the flesh, that lives far, far away from ordinary people's lives, should become a cult figure? Is it perhaps modern man's yearning for another unicorn, for the magical beast that lives in the never-never land over the horizon, or is it perhaps guilt or an easy option? Save the whale but keep on gobbling the chicken drumsticks and loins of lamb? It surely can't be a real concern that the species might become extinct, can it? If it were, would there not be a 'Save the medicinal leach!' or 'Save the British natterjack toad!' poster in every street? Romanticism undoubtedly plays a large part and, being a subjective quality, romanticism is by definition illogical.

Where exploitation may pass into plain cruelty we still seem to manage to fudge the issue. We are quick enough to apply anthropomorphic phrases – 'If I were a dog I know I'd feel . . .' – and thereby assume some strong similarities between the nervous system, anatomy and function of the senses in the naked ape and in other animals. Zoology would bear out that view. Pain, consciousness, unconsciousness, shock and reflex: they undoubtedly seem to exist in other species besides man. Isn't the eye of the octopus so similar to our own? Yes, but what about the millions of fish which we haul out of the water each year, many with metal hooks embedded in their throats, and which are allowed to 'drown' slowly in air? Lobsters: how many are killed before boiling? Frogs' legs and turtle soup: two more dishes that combine cruelty with every swallow.

It is interesting, too, how we select our arguments concerning cruelty. Anti-circus campaigners talk of animals being trained to perform 'unnatural' behaviours, like elephants pirouetting on their hind legs. Such criticism is rarely levelled at the 'circus' of dressage horses where animals also perform totally unnatural acts. But then, teaching one's dog to 'die for the queen' isn't natural, nor is much of the life style of Homo Sapiens Britannicus.

Some people regard certain areas of our exploitation of animals as being cruel in the sense that they 'degrade' animals, and one often hears the word 'degradation' applied to zoos and circuses. The definition of degradation is 'lowering in honour, estimation, character or quality'. If the correct and proper plane of animals is in the wild state, are not then all animals in captivity, wild or domesticated, degraded to some extent? Or could one not argue that lowering of esteem and honour is essentially in the eye of the beholder, in man? If so, does not exploitation of animals become a subjective quality of the exploiter – man? If, as seen some years ago on television from the London Palladium, two chimps dressed as boy and girl amuse the audience and bring the house down when the 'little boy' peeks into the knickers of the 'little girl', can we say that the animals are degraded? In the eyes of the audience, perhaps. But in enjoying such a spectacle, is it not the audience which shows itself to be degraded?

In the area of outright physical cruelty, there are areas when we still try to wriggle on the moral hook. British holidaymakers to Palma or Valencia flock to bullfights during the holiday season. They still trot out various potted rationalisations. Fox-hunters, hare-coursers, otter- and stag-hunters do the same. Beyond all that lies a darker, more secret world, where illegal blood sports like badger-baiting, dog-fighting, and cock-fighting still exist. Here one assumes that the apologists, if they have any apologia to make, would fall back on the 'dominion of man over the mere machines' argument.

There is yet another side to the relationship. It is poles apart from the factory farmers, the hunters and the coursers. This is the domain of the 'animal fanatics', some of whom would claim nothing less than equality for lesser creatures. Recently one gets the impression that the 'animal rights' movement has become increasingly vocal and militant, in both Britain and America. A religious attitude to animals is now being followed by a distinctly political thrust. Animal liberation front jargon is redolent of Red Brigade propaganda and animals seem to be pigeon-holed by many radicals along with underprivileged, exploited, *human* classes. Vegetarianism, Ban the Bomb and Women's Lib are apparently natural bed-fellows now for Animal Rights. But is it right to impose vegetarianism on dogs? Is that not political exploitation?

Just as dotty about animals but of a totally different political hue are the folk who literally seem to love animals at least as much as, if not more than, humans. For these the expensive veterinary hospitals, beauticians, holiday homes and pet cemeteries exist. Whether it is morally right for a country to be able to provide the pets of wealthy or well-insured people with filled teeth, advanced eye operations and plastic surgery, when humans in the third world still go blind or die because of the lack of simple drugs that can be found in any vet's surgery or RSPCA clinic in Britain, is a question worth pondering.

And what of the future? I suppose I am a sort of pessimist, for I see us passing from an age of an earth full of a variety of living creatures, to the irresistibly polluted earth of plastic and synthetics and microchips where our descendants will watch the videos of the 'old times' of Attenborough among gorillas and polar bears and the like and miss those extinct species as little as we feel deprived nowadays by the non-existence of the dodo or Steller's sea cow. Man, I believe, will always opt for the things that give him his creature comforts – oil, power, electronics – even though animals will die out one by one. A

124

few concrete 'zoos' will exist. There will be nuclear-shelter-trained pets of some sort. Then, after the holocaust, only a few radiation-resistant species will hang on. The age of the cockroach will dawn, insects will people the earth and the age of man and the myriad other furry and feathered species will be as gone as the age of the dinosaurs. That is evolution, unavoidable and completely natural.

And where does the poor old zoo vet fit in all this? For me I think the issue crystallises into the fight against suffering and pain. Disease – dis-ease – and pain are distortions, are evil. Whether they occur in a mouse or a man they represent the same distortion. The battle, the challenge, the fascination is in combatting these distortions. That, as I see it, is my job. I have written the last few paragraphs on a wet and stormy night shortly after returning from Chessington where I had been called to deal with an emergency in an animal that I had never previously operated upon. It was a mara, or Patagonian cavy, that delightful and gentle giant guinea-pig from South America. Somehow it had fractured a foreleg and with the aid of Ginger, the head keeper, and a big dose of ketamine anaesthetic I fitted it up with a plaster of Paris cast. After twenty-five years in the profession it was my first mara emergency. In the relief of pain and the mending of bodies there is always something new in wild animal medicine.

Surgery, although often of an emergency nature and always dramatic because of the exotic patients with their spectrum of anatomies, physiologies and varieties of disease, is not by any means as large a part of a zoo vet's work as medicine. Preventive medicine, often of a humdrum kind, saves a thousand times more animal lives than the more glamorous surgical procedures to remove tumours or mend shattered bones. Having said all that, I do relish the opportunity to take up scalpel and forceps and get to work. The physician can never be absolutely sure that his advice and prescriptions really are the cause of a cure; Nature truly is the best healer and wild animals have far stronger recuperative powers than do domesticated ones. But the surgeon can see exactly what he is doing and later witness the results, be they success or failure.

When I began working with exotic animals all those years ago, surgery on them was severely restricted by the lack of suitable anaesthetics for delicate, nervous or dangerous species. Even had the drugs been available, no simple means of delivery into the animal's body was to hand. Surgery could sometimes only be started when it was bound to be useless – when the patient was in extremis and too feeble and near death to put up any resistance. As I have described elsewhere,* the position changed rapidly in the late 'fifties. Pharmaceutical companies developed powerful and highly concentrated anaesthetics which could be injected by the other long-awaited invention, the flying dart, fired from a crossbow, pistol, rifle or blow pipe. By the mid-1970s the zoo vet could do anything to a gorilla, giraffe, walrus or porcupine that his colleague in general practice could do to dogs, cats, sheep and horses. And we arrived at the point where today I can honestly say that one of the safest and easiest of all animals to knock out is an adult elephant.

With anaesthesia under control, every sort of surgical technique could be made available when necessary in the world of wildlife. Hysterectomies on dolphins, vasectomies on over-productive tigers, the repair of hernias in elephants, Caesareans on zebras (I did the first one ever): it all could and did happen. Now, in several ways, exotic animal medicine leads the field in veterinary science. Not long ago, Andrew Greenwood and our assistant, Chris Furley, published a short paper on the use of the multi-million-dollar whole-body CAT scanner for visualising fungus infections in falcon lungs – and that is light years away from the arthritic elephant, Chota, that had to be euthanased by means of motor-cycle exhaust gases when I was a student.†

*See Zoovet, Doctor in the Zoo and Going Wild.
†See Zoovet.

Of course, it's the 'unusual' bits of surgery that tend to grab the interest of outsiders and particularly the journalists who find zoo stories and pictures perennial favourites for filling space and pleasing their readers. Such a case was Harry, the hornbill at Chessington Zoo. I can only imagine it began with a sort of itch, an itch at the tip of Harry's spectacularly large and yellow bill. It was a persistent itch and it came from within the tip. Harry did the obvious thing. He tapped his beak on his perch. But the itch did not go away. Irritated, Harry tapped some more. Still the itch persisted. It's bad enough for a primate with arms like you and me to have an itch right in the middle of one's back just out of reach of one's fingers. For Harry the itch was even more inaccessible, buried as it was beneath several millimetres of hard horn. There was only one thing for it: keep tapping the beak against the perch or anything else to hand that was solid. Surely the itch would fade sooner or later. It didn't. Instead, it turned into a very definite tickle. The hornbill, driven to distraction, hammered the troublesome appendage woodpecker-like against a log and so powerfully that a tiny piece of horn broke off the tip. Harry's itch, tickle, funny feeling or whatever a hornbill would have described it as, did not disappear.

The bird keeper became alarmed by the bird's incessant hammering away. It wasn't at all like Harry. When a bit more horn broke off the upper beak and Harry continued banging away, he told the head bird keeper. When Harry, otherwise quite norm.al and still enjoying his daily fruit salad and a dead white mouse, destroyed another inch of what is obviously the pride and joy of a hornbill – his horn bill – the head keeper consulted Lionel, the curator. 'Sounds like Harry's got an obsession,' he said, and called me.

Harry kept one wise eye firmly fixed upon me as I stood close to him where he sat on a branch in his aviary and went at the wood like a jack-hammer. He was doing considerable damage to himself – but why? Lionel grabbed Harry with the aid of a large butterfly net and held him clacking his beak indignantly while I examined him. There were no signs of infection or inflammation in the beak and I suspected that perhaps the small blood vessels deep in the centre of the bill or the nerve supply to the region might be the cause. Perhaps Harry had a local circulation fault or neuritis, the sort of thing that can cause tingling or numbness or pain in the extremities of humans. But it was only a guess: Harry wasn't talking and no-one had done any studies on 'chilblains of the beak' or such-like complaints in birds. 'Give him a complete change of environment, something to take his mind off things,' I told Lionel. 'Put him in another aviary.' I also prescribed some cortico-steroid and vitamin E to be given to Harry each day in a grape or piece of plum.

Harry lost no time after being moved in finding the hardest surfaces near to a suitable perch which would be ideal for the continuation of his dedicated self-mutilation. Within twenty-four hours he had smashed away almost one-third of his upper beak. The stump was damp with blood and there was a frantic look now in his orange and black eyes. He seemed to have an overwhelming hatred for his mouthpiece – if he had his way, it was all coming off. The hornbill didn't have any trouble feeding with upper and lower beaks of vastly different lengths, but scooped up his meals with his intact lower jaw, tipped back his head to swallow the goodies and then, when his stomach was full, returned at once to his day's (and night's) work of knocking his face to pieces.

When he reached the stage of possessing only one and a half beaks and was trying to squint down at the frayed and bloody stump with a crazy stare, no longer caring who was peering at him, I became very worried. Still I could find no cause for the bizarre compulsion. If there had been gangrene or pus in the beak I could have understood it, but the beak seemed normal enough. Harry had lived with it for seven years, so what was suddenly wrong with it now? I decided desperately to try tranquillising Harry. Doping birds, particularly for a long period, is a tricky business. I wanted to keep the hornbill eating, perching and behaving generally normally, but just dreamy enough to make him forget about the beak. I picked my perennial favourite – valium.

Valium isn't strictly a veterinary sedative, since vets have other drugs for controlling dogs, cats, pigs, cattle and other domestic animals, but for Andrew and me it is one of the safest and most important tranquillisers in exotic animals. Gorillas to gerbils, vicuñas to vampire bats – it works. The only problem is the dose rate. A chimp needs five times the amount necessary for a human adult. A Thomson's gazelle weighing perhaps seven kilos becomes dozy on twice the dose given to a human adult weighing say eighty kilos. Most importantly, we never found a species, however rare, in which valium produced bad effects. Compare that to say morphine, which can turn tigers and leopards into raving maniacs, or the promazine sedatives, which in certain antelopes produce a deadly rise in body temperature which may eventually end fatally by, as it were, 'poaching' the brain.

But what dose of valium to give Harry the hornbill? And in what form? I had never given the drug to any bird smaller than an emu before. In the end I opted for the human injectable solution of valium, but injected into one of Harry's grapes. 'Start with a tiny dose, say half a milligram three times a day,' I told Lionel, 'and work up slowly by increasing half a milligram per day. Don't, repeat don't, go beyond the point where he gets so 'high' that he falls off his perch!'

It didn't take Lionel long to discover that my dosage was far too low for Harry. Even on two milligrams three times a day, Harry hammered feverishly. 'Put him up by two milligrams a day,' I said. At five milligrams three times a day – enough to make you or me sleep soundly – Harry, who weighed around one kilo (including beaks or what was left of them), abruptly stopped his hammering and sat on a branch as placid as a hippy who's just fixed a good 'joint'. When he walked up and down we did notice a slightly inebriated weave and a barely perceptible droop of the upper eyelids, and when I went into him he positively beamed, letting me tickle his chest feathers and on one occasion nestling affectionately against my arm whilst taking a cherry from my fingers – and, incidentally, crapping affectionately in fashionable bottle-green and white down my jacket. I reduced the dose slightly but Harry still didn't hammer, and then set that as his daily regime for at least a month.

Now I had the next problem: horny beaks don't re-grow. How to replace the missing half? Harry without part of his upper beak just wasn't a hornbill and certainly could not be exhibited to the public who expect to see giraffes with four legs, elephants with two ears, kangaroos with one tail each and hornbills with a whole and proper set of matching horn bills. For repairing holes, splits and other defects in the horny toenails of elephants or hooves of giraffes I employ a special plastic compound made in Germany and similar to the stuff used by garages to fill holes in car bodywork. Consisting of a powder and a liquid catalyst which are mixed just before use, it is ideal for zoo chiropody. Perhaps I could use it to make a new half for Harry's upper beak, I thought. Anaesthetise him with ketamine, mix up the stuff and hey presto – apply with my artistic fingers an instant plastic beak. Sure, the plastic once set was of an unprepossessing dark grey colour, but some yellow paint should solve that little problem.

I gave Harry the ketamine, mixed powder and catalyst and, having cleaned up the stump of the mutilated beak, set to work like a latter-day Michelangelo. The result was somewhat lacking in sculptural genius because, designed as it was to repair holes and cracks in feet, the plastic once solidified was heavy as iron. Secondly, the smooth natural curves of a hornbill's beak eluded my fingers as they kneaded the grey amalgam into shape. The result was a grotesque, leaden-looking, knobbly beak that was so heavy that Harry was transmuted from a hornbill into a shoveller duck. He was weighed down by the monstrous thing and, but for the valium, would surely have redoubled his hammering when the anaes-

130

thesia wore off. Okay, so it didn't look much like a beak. Well, perhaps Henry Moore or Barbara Hepworth had more in common with my muse than Michelangelo. I removed the false beak and thought again.

I have always considered dentists to be more akin to plumbers than medical men and it was therefore not unnatural that I considered whether my next attempt at Harry's reconstruction should not be with the aid of dental surgery. Dentists are good at making crowns, fillings, bridges and the like – at falsifying nature, at persuading the artificial and inert to adhere to the living. Perhaps with their expertise in binding new strong materials to teeth, they could help me stick a passable, functional fake beak on Harry. I phoned the Eastman Dental Hospital in London, explained Harry's predicament and was connected at once with a most courteous professor of dental surgery. No problem: he would fit up Harry but, rather like a Savile Row customer, the bird would need to go in three times for measurement, fitting and final provision of the plastic beak. All I had to do was make sure that Harry was anaesthetised and dead to the world when he went down to the hospital on each occasion – dentists worry, understandably, about their fingers.

The techniques the hospital used for Harry were the same ones employed in constructing crowns that can resist the wear and concentrated pressures occurring in the human mouth, but magnified around two hundred times. The frayed bits of the bird's stump were removed and a mould of what was left carefully taken as for a set of dentures. Then a skilled dental technician moulded an extremely hard synthetic material around a virtually unbreakable central core of carbon fibre. As promised, at the third fitting the plastic beak – costing around £300 excluding veterinary fees – was fixed in place with dental cement. When Harry woke up this time he was fully equipped and beautiful once more.

The prosthesis was light as well as strong and the hornbill had no difficulty lifting his head. I stopped the valium drops and waited apprehensively to see what would happen. Nothing! The itch had apparently gone at last. Harry reverted to his old hornbill ways and seemed totally unaware that half his weight was inert plastic. He was put back into his own aviary and went on exhibition again. The visitors never knew what a bionic bird they were looking at – you couldn't see the join.

Other birds besides Harry have been re-beaked in this way. Toucans, pelicans and even budgerigars have received similar spare parts. And in Tampa, Florida, there is a macaw – a species that possesses a really powerful bite – with a complete bill of titanium steel. 'Jaws' really does exist, in the avian world at least. Beaks and hooves aren't the only bits of wild animals' bodies that I have had to send to the 'body shop'. Sometimes whole feet or even legs need substitution. Four-legged animals do considerably better after surgical amputation than two-legged ones, although in Holland there exists a very happy one-legged gorilla and a kangaroo that bounces along just as elastically on one leg as it did on two.

Birds which lose a leg for whatever reason – injury, gangrene, frostbite, intractable infection, tumours – may do OK, particularly if they are light, small, short-legged individuals. Bigger species with longer legs can find a sudden switch from biped to monoped highly inconvenient and often can't cope with the 'Hopalong Cassidy' role. Flamingoes, storks and cranes always seem to be getting into trouble with their pins. Providence designed their anatomy marvellously, with fine blood vessels, nerves and tendons all packed more ingeniously than the bits of a Japanese calculator into a slender, fragile tube. But providence overlooked the possibility of the wind blowing birds into fences, of foxes chasing them into a blind panic and of homo sapiens keeping them on unnatural hard surfaces and sometimes in places where the limbs are exposed to temperatures lower than speci-fied in the divine blueprint. Dud legs, as Providence now knows, tend to crop up with monotonous regularity. Am-putation is not difficult for the vet, but only Providence can grow new legs and so far hasn't shown any willingness to do so!

In the first days, when I worked mostly at Belle Vue Zoo in Manchester I had various types of false leg constructed for helping such feathered disabled. My first attempts with legs of wood and hinged wooden feet were better than nothing but had the disadvantage of being too heavy and unwieldy. On one occasion a newly fitted-up flamingo, trying to accommodate the strange, pink-painted device, waved it irresponsibly around and clouted a poor black swan that lived in the same pool smartly on the head. The black swan needed two weeks hospitalisation and treatment for severe concussion! Later designs were much more acceptable, built out of strong, ultra-light alloys with spring-loaded 'ankles' and leather 'feet'. The birds quickly learned to stand, walk, run and even mate on them. Of course I had to have them in for servicing once a quarter, and in winter attached a pad of tiny studs to the undersurfaces of the artificial feet to prevent skidding in birds that lived outside on pools that might ice over.

I have never been in favour of purely cosmetic dental surgery in exotic animals and do dental work, occasionally filling teeth, for sound health reasons only. Lions with the odd canine tooth or two sheared off during fighting don't usually suffer any ill effects and I leave them alone. There are a few lions in America with stainless steel crowns capping such damaged fangs. Although false teeth have been fitted to sheep to prolong their useful life, the problem of old age in elephants, when the last teeth are lost and the animal in the wild would starve to death, is dealt with most satisfactorily in the zoo or circus by the provision of lots of nourishing, soft and well-chopped grub that doesn't need chewing. On the infrequent occasions that I have an exotic patient which requires more complicated dental work in order to feed normally without pain or difficulty, I can call on my friend and colleague Andrees van Foreest in Holland, a vet who has specialised in veterinary dentistry. Say 'Aaaaahh', armadillo!

An extreme example of spare-part surgery gone wrong occurred a few years ago when I was in Germany, visiting a famous circus to treat an elephant with a paralysed trunk. While I was on the circus ground, the lady chimpanzee trainer, Señora Lapiz, asked if she could speak to me. After giving the elephant some injections, I went to the lady's caravan and was invited in to have a glass of schnapps. Señora Lapiz, the spitting image of the late Maria Callas, and I sat together on a couch in the luxurious lounge section. Between us, sipping orange juice from a paper cup and behaving like a proper little gent, sat a big male chimpanzee. From time to time between sips, he obligingly tried to pick my nose for me with one beefy black index finger.

'Problem eez thees, Doctor,' said the lady in a heavy Spanish accent. 'Pablo 'ere es not what 'e waz.'

'In what way? Is he ill?'

'No, no. I mean since 'e waz *castrado*.'

I don't approve of castration in animals such as chimpanzees and won't do the operation except for good medical reasons. 'Of course he's not what he was, Señora. He is minus his *cojones*!' I made the little joke in Spanish.

'Si, si! No, no! What I mean iz, since ze operation done by ze vet in Berlin he iz not 'imself. Before, 'e waz ze most active, most respected *hombre* in my show. All ze other chimps looked up to 'im as leader. Now 'e iz, I don' know 'ow you say it in English – bottom dog.'

'Well, castration does remove sexual drive. He can't be very macho without his . . .'

'Si, but I want you to do something.'

'But I can't put his testicles back in. Male sex hormone tablets might help a bit but . . .'

'No, I tell you my thinkin', Doctor. My friend is psychologist in Sevilla. 'E says it iz understandable like in humans who lose their . . . 'Ow you zay – it puts 'im down.'

'So?'

'Well, my friend zayz that humans who lose their . . . iz big

134

psychological shock. Hormones can only help a leetle. Main thing iz to give the man back a pair of . . .'

'But you can't replace testicles. There hasn't even been a testicle transplant in men yet.'

'No, no. I don' mean that. Ma friend zayz es a simple matter. You can do it, Doctor. Make Pablo think 'e 'az got his *cojones* back.'

'Think? How?'

'My friend zayz humans given two plastic *testiculos* feel all right again.'

'You mean you want two plastic what-nots put into Pablo's empty scrotum?'

'Si, exactly.'

There's always something new in a zoo vet's life. 'But chimpanzees don't think like humans, Señora. They are much less sophisticated mentally.'

'I don' know so much Doctor, but eef ze other chimps zee him with two big . . .'

'No, I'm sorry, Señora. I cannot do it.'

'Can't, Doctor, or won't?'

'No, I won't, Señora.'

The chimp trainer's face clouded over and she crossed her arms tightly under her ample bosom, thrusting it aggressively upwards. Pablo the eunuch sniffed and looked at me curiously. 'Okay, *vale*, Doctor.' The trainer's tone was now openly contemptuous. 'I'll get a good friend of mine, a *veterinario* who iz a real chimpanzee expert to operate. You obviously don' know nothing 'bout chimpanzee psychology. Good afternoon!' She stood up. Pablo gave me a back-hander to the solar plexus as I also got to my feet. Gasping for air, I opened the door and staggered down the steps.

Three months later, I was at the circus again; the elephant had regained almost totally the use of its trunk. To my surprise, the chimp trainer again asked to see me. 'She's had it done, you know,' confided the elephant man as I took a final blood sample from the elephant's ear. 'Had new balls put in the chimp. A pair of plastic whoppers big as duck eggs!' He chuckled and made an unprintable remark.

'I wonder what she wants me for this time,' I said. I found out soon enough. Pablo was sitting on the couch again when I entered the caravan. He looked morose and was sucking half-heartedly at an orange ice-lolly. Between his thighs I espied a piece of masculine anatomy of generous proportions.

'Good morning Doctor. I want you to zee Pablo. Like I told you, I've 'ad 'im done. Very good vet, very expensive.' The chimp trainer didn't offer me any schnapps this time.

'Is it working?' I asked.

'I theenk so. But it's early yet. Ze operation was only a month ago.'

'And what is your problem, Señora?'

'I theenk zere is some irritation een ze place of ze operation, where ze stitches were. Maybe you can geev me some cream?'

I went over to Pablo and bent down to look at his reconstructed codpiece. The scrotum was certainly causing irritation, but more than that, it was inflamed and weeping round the operation scar. Indeed, the scar itself appeared to be breaking down in parts. 'Señora,' I said after prodding the part and getting a painful clip to my ear from the chimpanzee, 'this is more than mere irritation. I think the plastic balls are producing a reaction and being rejected.'

'Impossible! Ze doctor said zis plastic ees same as used for making plastic hip joints.'

'Nevertheless, I think the body doesn't like them. I'll give you some anti-inflammatory ointment but the balls should be removed. It simply doesn't work.'

The chimp trainer did a mini-flamenco dance round the confined space of the caravan, spitting a stream of vitriolic Spanish. 'You are jealous, Doctor, you don' know nothing,' she hissed when the instant folkloric demonstration came to an end: 'Gi' me your ointment zen. Ez only irritation after ze stitches. And Pablo keeps 'is balls!'

Two weeks later I received a clipping from a German

136

newspaper, kindly sent by the elephant man. Some cub reporter had really gone to town over the story of an incident that had occurred during the previous evening's performance at the circus. 'Halfway through the chimpanzee act,' it read, 'the audience were amazed to see a chimpanzee lay two large eggs.' After 'giving birth' the 'mother' had continued unconcernedly participating in the repertoire of tricks. The article was headlined: 'MIRACLE CHIMP EXPECTING CHICKS!'

Nature, as is her way, had finally completed the rejection process used for ridding the body of objects which it recognises as foreign. What can be done with metal and synthetics in certain places cannot be done everywhere and without regard to certain physiological criteria. Pablo, I'm sure, would feel himself twice the man without the burden of his two 'eggs'. And Señora Lapiz still owes me ten Deutschmarks for the ointment.

8 Whale Doctor

The eyes of Kim, the Antibes killer whale, began to improve after the chloramphenicol injections and for a time my gloomy forebodings about his condition lightened. He seemed happy in the hospital pool where he was regularly visited by Martin Padley, Michael Riddell or some other member of the marine-land staff throughout the day. I, too, would spend half an hour with him as often as possible, plopping into the water beside him, paddling round his great body, stroking his flippers with my toes and talking to him. When he had had enough of our company he would give us a firm knock with his nose or politely show his teeth. Then it was time to climb out of the pool and let him take up his position by the massive metal door that separated him from the main pool, close behind which Betty and her two attendant dolphins would lie most of the time communicating to him in their secret language and, I suppose, doing their best to cheer him up in 'cetaceanese'.

But the regular blood analyses were not encouraging. The level of red cells was appallingly low, the antibody proteins remained high and now suddenly a new fault was observed: the tests for kidney function showed that these vital organs were in trouble. Everything in Kim's body seemed to be breaking down and Andrew and I began to talk of the possibility of imminent multi-organ failure. Every day, pints of French anti-anaemia liquid were injected into Kim's food fish and we made sure he had massive extra supplements of iron, trace elements, vitamin C and folic acid along with his usual vitamins. But nothing made any impression on the now thin and watery blood. As, years before, I had desparately tried to arrange a blood transfusion for Cuddles at Flamingo Park

138

when he suffered a massive intestinal haemorrhage,* so again I began to consider the possibility of taking a gallon or two from another killer whale. After all, on this occasion I had another whale to hand.

When I raised the matter with Michael he was understandably lukewarm about turning Betty into a blood donor, but typically said he'd go along with a transfusion attempt if I really thought there was a realistic chance of doing some good. 'How the hell are you going to get the gallons you need without stressing Betty by keeping her far too long out of the water?' he asked. A belligerent and excitable whale when put on the bottom of the pool, Betty was, as we knew from bitter experience, prone to overheating as well as to making dangerous sideways snaps at folks' legs. She wasn't playing either: if any of those snaps connected it wouldn't be a few nicks in one's skin through a torn wet suit but rather an instantaneous amputation. And to get blood, we'd obviously have to work as close as possible to her.

When I talked about gallons of blood, wasn't I anyway being terribly imprecise as to what was really necessary? Accurate calculations were essential. Aquatic animals have, as part of their adaptation to life in the water, much bigger blood volumes than terrestrial animals. Ducks, for example, have more blood than hens, and diving birds such as puffins more than non-diving species. The same goes for marine mammals, and radioactive iodine experiments on killer whales had shown that 10% of their body weight is blood volume compared with 8.5% in humans although some dolphins have as high as 15% and young elephant seals reach an amazing 20%. It worked out that in order to bring Kim's blood above the minimum level at which transfusions are ordered in anaemic human patients, he would need no less than sixty gallons of blood – almost exactly what I calculated Betty's total blood volume to be! So what about just giving some blood, as much as Betty could safely spare?

*See *Zoovet*.

My next task was to consider whether the blood of the two animals was compatible. Blood groups don't only occur in man. Bottle-nosed dolphins have several groups and at least two groups have been identified in fin and sperm whales. But nothing was known about killer whales although the probability was that they existed and would therefore be of crucial significance in any transfusion attempt. I decided to do the basic test, the only one open to me, of cross-matching Kim's and Betty's blood. This simply meant observing under a microscope how drops of blood taken from each of the two whales behaved when mixed together. I took two phials of blood to the local hospital laboratory and asked for the test to be set up. It didn't take a minute. When the samples were mixed on a square of smooth white tile, the formation of large clumps of red cells was quickly apparent even to the naked eye. No doubt about it: Kim's and Betty's blood definitely did not get on together. Even a pint or two of Betty's blood injected into Kim's system would cause serious and possibly fatal effects.

So ended all thoughts of transfusion, but while it had been a live issue I had spent much time pondering on how to physically extract large quantities of blood from a whale. After the failure of the cross-matching, this eventually led to a new line of thought. I had heard of a unique form of therapy being used in Germany on human patients which entailed the withdrawal of a quantity of blood from the body, treatment of it by ozone gas and then return of the blood into the patient's circulation. This ozone therapy was being credited with excellent results in various types of infectious disease and certain blood cancers. No-one seemed clear how it worked exactly, although ozone is a powerful killer of microbes. But with the potentially poisonous ozone gas only being applied to the blood outside the body, the procedure seemed safe to me.

One of the pioneers of ozone therapy of human disease in Germany was my friend Dr Ferdi Wurms, brother of Fritz Wurms, Director of the safari park at Stukenbrock. Dr Wurms and I had often met at Stukenbrock and discussed common areas of medical interest; brought up in a 'zoological' family, he was as much at home with the problems of sick animals as of sick people. I decided to ring him to see what he thought about trying ozone therapy on Kim. 'I've got a bull killer whale with what I believe to be a chronic focus of infection. How do you feel about coming down to Nice with the ozone machine and us having a try at washing his blood?'

'As soon as I finish my clinic this afternoon,' he replied, 'I'll be on my way. The maker of the ozone machines has a private plane, and I'll get him to fly me and all the gear down.'

Although it was April, the weather was bitterly cold on the Côte d'Azur. The wind howled down from the snow-covered Alps that seemed in the crystal-clear air of early evening to rise straight out of the orchards, cypress groves and red-tiled roofs behind the marineland. As I waited for Dr Wurms' plane to arrive, I worried again about the procedure. Perhaps I'd asked the German down on a fool's errand. Blood-sampling whales where a mere seven or ten millilitres is enough for a host of laboratory tests is one thing; pumping out litre after litre of blood and then pumping it back in again is something else. How long could I safely keep Kim dry on the bottom of a hospital pool? Would he lose patience and start flailing his tail around, dislodging the vital tubes? Could I find and connect with a big enough blood vessel that would provide a decent rate of flow? If clotting occurred in the needles, cannulas, tubes or whatever, how much damage would I inflict by multiple re-insertions? I realised that I'd have to use the tail veins. Only four of them would be big enough for the job so I would have only four chances.

Dr Wurms and Herr Felgner, the ozone machine maker, arrived on schedule with loads of equipment and, as is always my practice, we went straight to work. It was dark by the time Kim's pool was completely drained and the big whale was comfortably lying on thick pads of plastic foam which Martin and his team of trainers had slipped under his body just before the last few inches of water were pumped out. Banks of specially rigged floodlights illuminated the scene. The steadily dropping temperature and frosty wind were ideal for the whale. There was no chance of him overheating in such conditions, but for us in our motley assortment of dress – wet suits, swimming trunks, old jeans and wellington boots – it was increasingly unpleasant. My hands were soon numb from the spray of icy water which was continually hosepiped over the whale's body to assist the cooling process. Placing the tubes into the veins was going to be tricky.

All the instruments were taken down into the pool: oxygen cylinders, the ozone machine itself, dozens of blood transfusion bottles, black plastic tubes of every thickness by the yard and hundreds of sterile needles, including some that looked like miniature drainpipes. 'How much blood do you think we need to draw off for treatment?' I asked Ferdi Wurms.

'Well, going by comparison with humans, I would say we should wash at least thirty litres – seven gallons.'

'Any idea how long that would take?'

'In a man, ozone washing of one litre, which is normally all we need to do, takes maybe twenty minutes. The machine draws out the blood into the flasks by suction, then the blood is shaken gently to mix it with a known volume of ozone that is produced electronically in the machine by conversion of oxygen, and then the blood is sent back into the circulation through the same tube and needle under positive pressure. Easy.'

'But thirty litres would take ten hours by that reckoning.'

The German pulled his anorak hood close around his face and smiled gently. 'Yes. And that's if the tubes and needles don't get blocked up by coagulation.'

Ten hours on the bottom – if all went smoothly! Still, La Soeur had said all that time ago that everything was going to be all right, even if nothing had happened at the hour she had specified. Maybe the ozone machine was the 'three things'.

142

After all there was the machine itself, the oxygen cylinder and the glass flask.

I was clutching at straws. 'OK. Let's get started,' I said. 'The first thing is to plant a big needle securely into a big vein' (something that had never been done before in a killer whale). 'Put the heaviest net we have over the narrow part of the tail and have four men sit on it at each side.' The net with its chain and lead weights must have weighed about four hundred-weights. With eight men in addition, maybe, just maybe, it would be enough to stop me being smashed in the face by the tail flukes if Kim objected to being the guinea-pig in this rare experiment.

When the tail stock seemed reasonably secure, I knelt down by the flukes and signalled for Wurms to move the equipment ready for connection. I injected some local anaesthetic into the skin over the main blood vessel on the upper surface of the tail and then, shivering from the cold, I took a needle five inches long and as thick as a pencil. Sucking in my breath and gritting my teeth, ready for all hell to break loose, I stabbed it into the numbed area. Killer whale tail flesh is as tough as green wood; it has to be to form such a powerful paddle. I gave a grunt and pushed with all my strength. The thick needle moved on and suddenly I was blinded by a bright red curtain – I had struck oil. The needle had entered at first attempt the central artery.

Wiping my face and blinking through the gore, I saw a powerful jet of bright red arterial blood spurting out of the needle. 'Connect up!' I shouted.

Ferdi Wurms moved in with a plastic tube and attached it to the needle. At once blood raced up the tubing and began to fill the big glass bottle held by Martin. The ozone machine hummed. I could smell the characteristic 'seaside' smell of ozone in the chilly air. Normally veins, not arteries, are used for sampling and injection but for this technique either would do. With the circuit set up, I sat back on my haunches and watched. Kim didn't seem to have noticed a thing; he was in his most co-operative mood. I watched the piston on the machine move as it sucked air out of the receiving bottle. Herr Felgner twiddled knobs and adjusted the ozone concentration. Martin seemed mesmerised by the rising tide of red in the bottle that he held and shook gently as Ferdi Wurms instructed. I looked for signs of clotting in the plastic tubing and the filter of the bottle itself but couldn't see any. Thank God or, as Michael later suggested with a certain ecclesiastical wittiness, Saint Januarius, that whales and all other cetaceans have a pro-longed blood-clotting time (the average clotting time for bottle-nosed dolphins is three-quarters of an hour).

Sure enough, we had a litre of blood within about ten minutes. When the bottle was full, ozone was pumped in and the blood/ozone mixture was gently shaken while the machine was reversed and began to push the blood back down the tube and into the artery. As soon as the bottle was empty, Wurms and Felgner began the cycle again and blood once more surged up into the bottle. From time to time samples of blood were extracted from the system and taken by one of the trainers on his motor-cycle to the hospital laboratory a couple of miles away for oxygen level analysis. The technicians and doctors there, bless their hearts, have always been happy to provide us with a round-the-clock service 365 days a year. None of the National Health Service mentality – 'Love to help you, Doc, but there'd be bloody hell to pay if the NUPE shop steward got to know we were handling animal blood' – that we have some-times encountered in Great Britain when handling emergen-cies in the middle of the night and far away from our usual veterinary laboratories at Newmarket and Weybridge.

At the third filling of the bottle I noticed that the blood seemed to be flowing more reluctantly. 'Some coagulation developing in the system,' said Dr Wurms. 'Check the needle.'

I disconnected the plastic tube from the needle in Kim's tail. The gout of bright blood that pulsated up towards me was as strong as ever. 'It must be in the tubes or bottle,' I said. Wurms prepared a new unit and we changed over. Everything ran smoothly once more.

144

The cold intensified and, with all of us clustered round the whale being relatively immobile except for Martin who continued his bottle-shaking, cramps and numbness began to set in. 'I must get something warmer,' I muttered through chattering teeth to Michael. 'The cold is coming straight through wet suit, two sweaters and a duffle coat!'

Michael is probably the best 'fixer' in the whole of France, and he disappeared to return after a few minutes with half a dozen bottles of Vin du Var and a lady's astrakhan fur coat. 'Some old bird left this here a few weeks ago,' he said. 'Try and squeeze into it.' Somehow I managed to stretch the fur coat over all my other garments. It did the trick. 'Must be worth the best part of ten thousand francs,' said Michael, 'but she really ought to have collected it before now.' At each of the following changes of tube and bottle the exquisite astrakhan got a bloody drenching, but I was soon as warm as toast. Michael kept the Vin du Var flowing.

The hours passed by and Kim remained utterly placid. I checked his heart and respiration, felt for 'hot spots' on his forehead, flippers and flukes, smelled his breath: everything was good and stable. We changed ten litres, then fifteen, twenty and twenty-five. The pile of discarded transfusion units on the pool bottom mounted steadily.

At last, and with the original needle still firmly in place and running as freely as it had at the beginning, the final weak litre was washed in the ozone and returned to the whale's circulation. With a sigh of relief I removed the needle and slapped on a pad of cotton wool. 'Get all the gear out of the pool and begin filling up,' I said wearily.

Dawn was breaking over the Mediterranean and the caked blood on my astrakhan coat was frozen and glistening. 'You look like a damn' great Black Forest gâteau,' Martin remarked.

We breakfasted as is the custom after nightwork at Marineland Côte d'Azur on whole ungutted mackerel (the same fish that the whale and dolphins get), grilled over a wood fire set in a rusty old wheelbarrow and accompanied by fresh baguettes of bread, lemons and red Provencal wine. Then, leaving one man to watch over the whale as he floated up with the steadily rising water, we went off to snatch a few hours sleep. At least we had proved that transfusion and similar techniques involving the movements of large quantities of blood in giant mammals were technologically possible.

The ozone therapy didn't produce any ill effects on Kim. With his pool full again he even seemed a little chirpier and did some upside-down swimming, a cheerful sign in killer whales. I waited two days before taking my first blood sample after the treatment. The results of the analysis were amazing – the level of antibody protein in the blood had dropped steeply. For the first time since he fell ill, the graph that plotted his internal battle with infection showed a turn for the better. 'We must repeat the treatment,' I told Michael excitedly. 'This could be the answer to all our troubles.' Wurms and Felgner flew down from Germany again a few days later and in now much milder weather conditions we washed Kim's blood a second time.

We also made an heroic attempt at x-raying his chest with a powerful industrial set that could penetrate metal. It entailed covering the whole of one side of his body with x-ray film and the conversion of an ice-cream kiosk into a temporary dark room. Sadly, the radiographs were useless and showed nothing; the whale's dense tissues in his broad trunk scattered the x-rays in all directions.

More depressingly, in the days following the second ozone therapy, there was no further dramatic improvement in the blood sample and within a month the antibody levels started to rise once more and Kim stopped accepting fish altogether. My tests showed serious kidney failure now: a human or a chimpanzee with an analysis as bad as that would not be expected to live more than a few days unless put on to an artificial kidney machine. Michael, typically, actually made enquiries about hiring such equipment but it was hopeless – the same problem of the massive blood volume of a killer whale confronted us. Human kidney machines are capable of treating an animal containing a mere eight pints of blood in its body. Kim would have needed to be linked up to two dozen kidney machines simultaneously!

Because of the impossibility of forcibly getting anything down the whale's throat, I wondered how I might flush his system through with fresh water; stomach tubing was out of the question. A scientist in Denmark had recently proved that porpoises, contrary to what we had believed up to that time, could absorb water through their skins, a frog-like facility which was most unexpected in marine mammals. Perhaps killer whales too could 'drink' through their skins. 'Let's fill up Kim's pool with pure tap water,' I said to Michael.

He looked aghast. 'But it has always been said that dolphins and whales in fresh water get skin disease and have difficulty with buoyancy.'

'The buoyancy idea is nonsense. As for the skin, well, two or three days won't do any harm. Even if it does peel a bit, so what? We're in big trouble. Cosmetic matters can wait.'

Michael reached for the phone. 'Get the fire brigade,' he told his secretary. 'We'll need them to pump in from the hydrants. Oh, and give the Fire Chief my compliments and tell him it's the mad professor from England again. There'll be the usual free dinner and champagne for him and his crew if he can get it done this evening.'

The Chef des Pompiers in Antibes had helped out magnificently on numerous occasions in the past when we had had water problems, even providing fire engine escorts when animals were being transported from the airport to the marineland. 'I am ze 'ead of all zings to do wiz water in ze 'ole area, professor,' he told me when we first met at the opening of the marineland. 'Dolphins, whales, zay leeve in ze water so voila! It iz my job just like fires and rescues to look after zem, n'est-ce pas?'

'Oui, ah oui,' I had replied. 'And maybe, professor,' the

Chief had carried on, 'you will train me some dolphins for me to 'elp bring back ze corpses of drowned people.'

'That is your province also?'

'Mais naturellement, professor – everyzing to do wiz water.'

The firemen duly arrived and Kim's salt water was changed for fresh. Within twenty-four hours the beneficial effect of the fresh water was clearly to be seen in the whale's blood. I arranged for Kim to be kept alternately in three days fresh and three days salt water from them on. The fire brigade would be eating and drinking well that spring!

The kidneys were still not functioning normally, however, and I had to find some more specific line of therapy. Pills and potions were out; Kim still wasn't eating. There was nothing among orthodox injectable drugs that I felt might be beneficial. I had already dabbled in the highly unorthodox in this case what with the Antoiniste sister and the magical ozone machine, so perhaps there would be no harm in trying herbal remedies. Many 'orthodox' drugs like digitalis, atropine, strychnine and the antibiotics are strictly of herbal origin. Although I was not familiar with the broad field of herbalism which claims to provide remedies for the whole spectrum of ailments human and veterinary, I consulted the French pharmaceutical tomes where orthodox and unorthodox medicines and their applications are listed alongside one another. Continental physicians are not as toffee-nosed as their British counterparts over so-called alternative medicine. I found an injectable liquid compounded from the fresh leaves of a plant with a Latin name, *Cynara scolymus*. At least such vegetable extracts should not do any harm, even if they did no good. I ordered two thousand bottles of the stuff – and probably made a significant contribution to the balance sheet of the little pharmaceutical company that manufactured it.

Martin and his men began injecting Kim with the herbal kidney preparation, which looked and smelled rather like Coca-Cola, every eight hours. Kim was by now very thin and his breath had become foul-smelling. And, like everything else

148

to do with whale medicine, the unpleasant odour was big: it was detectable many yards away and this of course in the open air.

Although otherwise his breathing continued to be normal with never a sign of cough and there was nothing I could hear through his mighty chest wall with my stethoscope, I began increasingly to suspect that Kim's hidden focus of infection might lie in the lungs. I still stuck firmly to the diagnosis of a chronic thick-walled abscess in soft tissue despite increasing scepticism on the part of the French vets and laboratories who opted for leukaemia, and despite La Soeur with her 'grille'. There had even been a gratuitous diagnosis by a man with a 'black box' who literally stole a few drops of Kim's blood from our small laboratory in the marineland itself and phoned us to say that his wondrous machine had without a shadow of a doubt indicated a severe liver disease in the whale. For a few thousand francs he would be prepared to mix his own remedy.

Despite all the doubts as to whether my line of reasoning on Kim's illness was correct, Michael Riddell, Andrew Greenwood and Martin Padley, who had followed the grim saga every inch of the way and with whom I discussed each of the innumerable laboratory results and dissected my conclusions, gave me unwavering support and agreed with my general thesis. If only we could get at the secret fortress of germs and wipe them out! The trouble with abscesses is that even with antibiotic treatment they usually need draining ultimately. Either they burst or are lanced. But you can't lance something unless you know where it is. Anyway, open-chest surgery on whales was out of the question. We have one anaesthetic machine in Great Britain that can keep a dolphin breathing while its chest is opened but the apparatus big enough to ventilate Kim simply doesn't exist.

The strain of round-the-clock nursing of the big whale week after week and month after month showed in the faces of the marineland staff. Night work, cold water, the physical strain of pushing and pulling heavy equipment and the whale himself, the tedium of long hours standing with their arms extended,

149

holding an intravenous bottle or an oxygen lance, the discomfort of crouching or kneeling in a fixed position holding a needle or a tube at a precise angle: all this on top of the day's regular routine work of preparing the marineland for thousands of visitors, cutting the fish and presenting the shows going on as usual seven days a week. The worst thing that insidiously sapped us all was the feeling that we were, for all the occasional minor triumphs and apparent moments of success, losing the war. Kim was fighting hard but was it hard enough?

Chronicling all this, as in the earlier books that I wrote, I record events as they actually occurred. The American publishers of my first autobiographical volume, *Zoovet*, asked me to 'soften' several of my stories to ensure that there were always happy endings, less gore and pain and an abundance of 'Ohh-ahhs!' as the little tiger cub or elephant or giraffe takes up its bed and walks. I have always resisted this approach. The care of wild animals isn't all dewy eyes and plaudits: it is rough, tough and so often depressingly, frustratingly a failure. It isn't all funny or easy – and it is best told as it is.

Phone calls at 3 am for me invariably mean trouble, so when I picked up the receiver one morning a week after the start of the herbal mixture, I was ready for some grim tidings of death or disaster. Michael's voice, however, was far from sombre. 'He's begun to eat again!' he announced before I could complete 'Bagshot 75. . . '. 'The night watchman tried him as usual ten minutes ago and he gobbled five kilos of mackerel and is asking for more.'

Kim was doing yet another of his displays of medical brinkmanship. 'Get Martin out of bed,' I said. 'Ask him to take blood at once and have the lab run the usual series of kidney function tests.' By breakfast time the results were in and we had the stunning reason for the whale's remarkable improvement: the kidneys were working perfectly normally again! I ordered the vegetable injections to be continued another month and telephoned the local bookshop to order a copy of *Culpeper's Compleat Manual of Herbs*.

150

Acupuncture in giraffes, white magic in the case of Cuddles the killer whale* and now herbal remedies for Kim! 'What next?' Hanne asked as I opened the morning mail. (From one extreme to the other: there was a letter from a lady in New York who had a paralysed brown mouse. Could I please advise? I sent her a note and a tiny bottle of medicine to put in its water.) 'Chiropractic for crocodiles?'

'Why not? Or maybe a spell in the waters at Baden Baden might be just the thing for sick whales,' I replied.

Kim's kidneys never faltered again and the foul smell from his blow hole soon cleared with the spraying of anti-fungal aerosols down the nostrils when he breathed – a tricky job. The blow hole opens and shuts quickly and is designed to keep out strong seas, let alone stuff squirted in by human beings. It needed a steady hand and good reflexes to deliver the jet into the hole which opened only at irregular and lengthy intervals.

The anaemia and high antibody levels continued as bad as ever, though, and he was down by now to half his normal weight, a sad, snake-like shadow of his former plump and glistening self. In a desperate effort to knock out the elusive bugs with something that could penetrate the less accessible areas of the body, I was now using the very expensive anti-tuberculosis antibiotic, rifampicin. It is rarely used for diseases other than TB but it can destroy a wide range of bacteria and it finds its way into the chronic well-walled nodules of tuberculosis, so perhaps it could infiltrate the stronghold of my hypothetical encapsulated abscess. One of rifampicin's common and harmless side-effects in humans is the staining red of the urine, saliva and tears. Killer whales naturally produce copious syrupy tears as a protection against the friction of movement through sea water. Kim on the rifampicin looked like some horrific monster from a Hammer film, weeping and drooling 'blood'. Despite normal kidney function the whale's appetite began to fade again by March 1982. It finally stopped completely and on 3 April I received

*See Zoovet.

the phone call I'd always known deep down I'd receive one day: Kim had died peacefully during the night.

The Sunday airbus to Nice was full of jolly up-market holidaymakers and the moneyed English expatriates of Monte Carlo and Juan-les-Pins. Lady Docker was sipping champagne across the aisle and I sat next to Cary Grant, who politely offered me his cheese. He wasn't hungry, but neither was I. In the rack above, among all the Gucci handbags and fur stoles, was the Bag, full of scalpels, sample bottles and sharp saws. I caught a whiff of my formalin bottle cutting through the mists of 'Opium' and 'Rive Gauche'. When a passing stewardess wrinkled her nose and looked up, trying to locate the source of the smell as usual, I never let on – as usual.

Many miles from the sea, in the quiet Provencal countryside near Gap, there lives a knackerman who has a keen amateur interest in whales and has disposed of the carcasses of many of the cetaceans washed up on the coastline of France. In his processing shed I performed the autopsy on Kim, helped to the end by Michael and Martin. There was no 'grille', nothing untoward between stomach and intestine, no leukaemia, no cancer, no diseased liver. But an abscess as big as a sack of coal, with a tough fibrous wall an inch thick, lay deep in the right lung. If I had known for sure its size or precisely where it lay, if x-rays had been possible on an animal of such a girth, if I had had a special extra-long cannula made and pierced the abscess through the chest wall and drained it, Kim could have made it. If.

I sat on the terrace of the marineland at Palma Nova in Majorca eating thin wafers of *jabugo* ham and splitting a bottle of Valdepeñas with my close friend the director, Robert Bennett. We had finished the routine two-monthly inspection of all the animals and in an hour I had to catch the one o'clock Iberia flight to London. 'By the way, I've got a little present for you,' said Robert, pulling something out of his pocket, 'the first of a new line of up-market souvenirs we've had made for the coming season.' Onto the table between us he trickled a chain carrying an exquisitely moulded pendant of a leaping dolphin in solid silver.

While I was admiring the gift, a posse of English tourists swept by, making for the bar in search of tea or Sangria and shade from the burning sun. One lady, lobster-red and perspiring, saw the shining pendant and in an unmistakable Manchester accent said to the man walking beside her, harnessed like a brewer's draught horse in a mesh of photo-graphic equipment, 'Ay, Melvin, take a look at that. You can buy me one of those before we go back.'

'Right, luv,' replied the camera buff. 'Certainly, my dear.'

The incident at once recalled to my mind something which happened to another Melvin and his spouse six or seven years ago in the latter days of Manchester's Belle Vue Zoo.

The red-neck ostrich in Belle Vue was having one of his better days. Normally he was utterly bloody-minded and anti-social. He liked nothing better than terrorising his keeper, fluffing out his apologies for wings and trying to leap high enough to stamp down on the man's head. On occasions in the past he had managed to kick the keeper in the solar plexus and flatten him. He'd broken one of the fellow's fingers and chipped a vertebra in the triumphant dance that followed, up and down the keeper's prone body. But today was indubitably one of his good days. Maybe it was the unaccustomed blue of the Manchester sky and the silver sun peeping over the Ardwick Hippodrome or the sound of the rushing roller-coaster across the park, warming up for the start of the Easter season, that mellowed him. At any rate the ostrich – he of the fearsome countenance, red-rimmed eye and iron-hard beak – was, as I insist, in a better mood. He was unarguably milder, no more than cantankerous, crotchety and quibbling. He hadn't, it would seem, had anything to quibble at all morning. No-one had looked at him in the wrong way. No-one had given him the faintest excuse for a punch-up. It was a good day. Until the lady with the pendant came along.

She was to humans a good-looking bird (I cannot speak for ostriches) and she wore a silver mink coat, silver stiletto heels and a silver necklace and pendant. Behind her trailed the probable fount of all these goodies – a small, globular, harassed-looking gentleman in a camel coat and brown 'racing man's' trilby. The ostrich didn't care for, in fact positively resented, the way in which she and then he stopped in front of his paddock and proceeded without so much as a by-your-leave to stare at him. It ruined the ostrich's erstwhile comparative euphoria. He took immediate remedial action. Advancing smartly towards the gawking couple, he did his usual: whipped out his long red neck, opened the steely beak and snapped at the lady's silver pendant. With one gulp and a 'Yawk! Friggin' 'ell, Melvin, look what it's done to me!' the bauble was safely ensconced within the ostrich's gizzard. Honour satisfied, the ungainly bird turned away and stalked off, sniggering, I suspect, if indeed ostriches can snigger.

The encounter resulted in my being summoned by Matt Kelly, the head keeper, to do something. Silver-mink was doing her nut, he told me over the telephone, demanding the retrieval of her plundered pendant pronto. I drove down to the zoo and found Matt in an embattled position. He was standing by the ostrich paddock confronted by the silver mink lady who was giving him hell, the camel-coated gent who was looking even more harassed and mopping his brow and the red-neck ostrich who was looking for trouble. 'That effin' bird's got my pendant!' shrieked the silver mink. 'Gerrit back or I'll sue you!'

'Darling, I keep telling you it's not platinum, it's only silver plate. I bought it, I know. Let the bird keep it'. That was camel-coat.

'Well now, Oi'm sure Dr Taylor can help us here,' said Matt – passing the buck craftily as I arrived.

'I want my pendant back or I'll sue for assault, for theft, for grievous bodily whatever, for gross incompetence!' Silver-mink stamped her silver heels.

154

'Darling, cool it, my luv. I'll buy you another one, angel. It wasn't worth the sweat. Twenty nicker, as I live.' Camel-coat was looking as if he were about to break into tears.

'Shurrup, Melvin!' snapped silver-mink. 'You 'aven't got no effin' idea and no spunk.'

Camel-coat blew his nose and shurrup.

'I presume the red-neck snatched something,' I said diplomatically.

'Effin' right,' said silver-mink.

'It would seem so, Doctor,' said Matt in his lovely brogue. 'Taken the lady's pendant.'

'Want it back *now!*' snapped the lady.

'No go, I'm afraid,' I replied, 'but if its not been passed by the bird within seven days, then I might operate.'

'But . . .'

'Seven days,' I repeated loudly. 'Come back then, madam, and we'll have it one way or the other.'

The ostrich elected not to excrete the pendant in the usual way. A week went by and still the jewel was safely tucked away in its innards. I brought a portable mine-detector to the zoo and sure enough there was a positive pinging response over the crop area. An operation was unavoidable. With the deadline expired, I had Matt catch up the enraged bird and throw a sack over its head. Then I opened the crop under local anaesthetic. It was a simple matter to reach in and withdraw the pendant, looking surprisingly unaffected by long contact with digestive fluids. No sign of corrosion, tarnishing or verdigris. Silver-mink and camel-coat appeared on cue after I'd finished the operation. I handed her the pendant – 'With the ostrich's compliments,' I said.

'Ta very much,' replied silver-mink.

'I'm sorry that the bird has had to go through this,' muttered camel-coat. 'Really the pendant wasn't worth a light. But the wife . . .'

'Well, you've got it back now,' I butted in. 'No harm done.' The couple went out of Matt's office. 'Funny that such a cheapy didn't corrode at all,' I remarked to Matt after they had gone.

In the same instant the door opened and silver-mink darted back in. 'Psst! Melvin's gone for a pee. That pendant really is platinum, you know. *He* thinks it's silver plate and so it was, the one that he bought me, the schlepper. This one's identical, but in platinum – a present from a friend, a *very* good friend!' She winked, turned round and clicked out on her silver heels.

Matt and I looked at one another – for once both mute as ostriches.

'Dr Taylor come quickly, *please*. She's eaten all but one of 'er childer!' The lady on the other end of the telephone was sorely distressed, as well she might have been. Living in the Lancashire cotton town of Bury, in a drab, drizzle-grey triangle that had a brook blocked by bedsteads and tin cans as its base with the gas works, a derelict Wesleyan chapel and a willow-herb-covered rubbish-tip at its corners, Mrs Stansfield had always been one for exotic pets. A diminutive, rosy-cheeked widow, she had possessed the only loris I've ever seen taking the place of a fireside cat. And where others would keep a budgie, a parrot or perhaps a mynah bird, she preferred a one-winged flamingo that had been found to everyone's surprise on a local reservoir after surviving an encounter with a high-tension cable and then went on to recover from a subsequent amputation. It occupied most of the tiny bathroom of the house and fed from a soap-holder converted to hold a mash of beetroot, dried shrimp and dog meal. The bread-bin in her kitchen, lined with hay, was the kennel of an ancient hedgehog, blind from cataracts in both eyes, and there were two free-flying plum-head parakeets in the front room who had shredded everything from wallpaper to soft furnishings, from the books on the shelves to the music sheets on the upright piano. She adored and pampered them and they were as plump as dormice and arrogant as fighting cocks.

In a greenhouse in the back yard was the object of her present concern, a female six-banded armadillo that she had bought about a month earlier from an animal dealer in Manchester's Tib Street. It seemed to thrive well in the greenhouse and possessed a prodigious appetite for eggs, milk, tomato juice, minced meat and the occasional chunk of melon: good armadillo grub. Then, only twenty-four hours ago, she had telephoned me in high excitement to say that the armadillo had produced six tiny babies out of the blue! As the mother didn't seem to be caring for them very conscientiously, could I advise on a suitable milk formula for dropper feeding.

I had been surprised and delighted at the good lady's news. Armadillos often breed in captivity with up to twelve young in a litter which may all be identical dodecaduplets (if that is the correct word) of the same sex, formed by the splitting of one single fertilised ovum. Rearing them, even if their mother does her stuff, is not easy and normally few survive. As for artificial armadillo milk – I have been asked for even stranger things – I had suggested cow's milk in a two to one mixture with water plus a little glucose. Any weakly ones were to be given a few drops of neat protein hydrolysate hourly for the first day or two. I had made a note to go over to Bury as soon as I had the opportunity to see the unexpected sextuplets.

Now here she was again, utterly distraught. All had apparently gone wrong. Many animals will eat their dead or dying young, as if it were Nature's way of tidying up without wasting precious protein, but I had never come across an infanticidal armadillo; that was more like tigers, bears or wolves. Perhaps I should have advised her to separate mother and young, but armadillos are such gentle creatures – I never thought, damn it. I promised her I would go over at once and went out to my car.

It is rare enough to see armadillos in Lancashire, let alone newborn baby armadillos. I cursed our luck as I swung out of Woodhouse Lane and took the road over the moor towards Bury, lying under a mantle of smoke in the next valley. Mrs Stansfield's pink face was streaked with tears as she opened the door and led me through the hallway to the back yard. 'A reet bonny little beggar, Doctor, and so kindly. Why would she murdur all 'er childer?'

'Well, I can't say, but sometimes if a mother recognises some fault in her young, perhaps something we humans can't discern, she'll act that way.'

The armadillo, a grey rugby football, lay sleeping in a wooden box in one corner of the greenhouse. Armadillos are night people who spend most of the daylight hours dozing, and it was now early afternoon. I gently lifted out the curled-up animal and it began to wriggle in my hands as it roused. I couldn't see any armadillo baby left behind in the hay-lined box.

'Oh Doctor, she's et'n t' last one,' wailed Mrs Stansfield. 'All six babies in one day!'

'Just move the hay, Mrs Stansfield,' I said. 'Maybe it's got underneath.'

The armadillo's hard claws scrabbled irritably at my arm. Its owner bent down and began to rummage through the bedding. Almost at once she gave a shrill squeak. 'Ooh look, Doctor, you're reet. It is still here. Come on, me little bobby-dazzler.' Fiddling about with her fingers in the hay, she seemed to have some difficulty catching the infant but finally she straightened up and turned to me beaming, with the palms of her hands cupped together. 'A wick little bugger, Doctor, ah'll have to be careful not to drop it.'

Very slowly she began to open her hands and I looked in. I got a good view of the 'survivor'. Scurrying frantically over one calloused pink palm was a fat woodlouse.

There must have been dozens of such 'baby armadillos' if she'd hunted thoroughly through that greenhouse, all of them just the sort of toothsome live food that armadillos and other insectivorous mammals go searching for after dusk. Mrs Stansfield flushed with embarrassment when I explained. 'Aah well, Doctor,' she said, shuttling as she made me a cup of tea, 'I bet that's the first insect you've ever been called to look at, eh? Aren't I a one, eh?'

'It's not an insect, Mrs Stansfield, it's a crustacean, a relative of the lobster. And I have been called to deal with those before,' I said.

Mrs Stansfield seemed much relieved at hearing that. 'Ay well then, Doctor, that's all reet then, innit. I'm not so daft after all! Any road, when you've drunk up I'd like you to come and look at these snakes that I've got that I'm keeping in the airing cupboard.'

9 The Constipated Camel

The black camel stood beside the sun-bleached tent and did nothing. That was the trouble. The old Bedou sitting cross-legged on a rug just within the shadowed threshold of the tent door scratched his camel stick irritably in the sand and muttered to himself, 'Aiwa! This was indeed ill fortune.' The other camels, two dozen or so, were all lying down facing the midday sun, instinctively exposing as little of their skin surfaces to the blazing white heat as possible. As the sun moved they shifted their position with it to maintain the alignment and comfortably chewed their cud.

The Bedou didn't know why camels pointed at the sun in this way, undoubtedly had never even wondered how hairy animals like camels avoid over-heating in the desert environment and couldn't have guessed that pointing at the sun was only one of several clever tricks of Nature that they had up their sleeve. But he had lived and worked with camels since – since, it seemed, his mother weaned him. He rode racing camels when he was five years old. By the time he was seven he could throw a camel to the ground with an artfully wound rope in a trice and hobble it securely in but a few moments longer. He had drunk camel milk all his life and eaten camel meat at all the great festivals of the Mohammedan year. From his grandfathers and his father he had learned the ways of the camel and the limits to which the animal could be taken: ten days without food, twelve days without water. He knew that a camel can carry 120 to 220 kilos for twenty miles a day, that it has difficulty traversing ditches unless small enough to stride across, but that it is a good swimmer; he had seen them cross wadis filled with rushing water after a flash flood. He knew camels need five to ten minutes rest every hour when on the move in order to urinate – male camels pass water *very* slowly. Above all, he knew that the first sign a camel gives that he is being asked to do the impossible is often to drop down dead.

The Bedou had also inherited all the remedies for the illnesses from which his animals might suffer – bitter desert melons for tapeworms, sugar thrown into the eye to clear corneal ulcers – but even for him the black camel was a problem. It did nothing. For seven days it had not eaten, drunk nor passed a scrap of dung. It had refused fresh onions and lucerne brought from a distant souk. It had disdained even to sip the contraband Tunisian date liquor which he kept for just such cases in camels (as a devout Moslem he would never have dreamed of drinking the sweet alcoholic beverage himself). Rice bowls, mint tea, fermented eggplants, roasted camel spiders: he had pressed all these usually efficient pick-me-ups on the camel but to no avail. 'Aiwa! A misfortune indeed.' For the black camel was the favourite of her owner, the Ruler of the Arab state of Qatar.

'Perhaps it will be necessary to send for the animal doctor from Cairo who lives in Doha. Zehn, zehn, that would be best.' The old camel man spat on the sand and called to a boy in a ragged smock who was running gazelle-nimble up the slope of the nearest pale gold dune in pursuit of a runaway goat. 'Ali, leave it! Take the young one, Fatma, and ride down to the vizier's office. Tell him the black camel is sick. Ask him to radio Doha for the Egyptian doctor.'

The boy turned and ran back down the slope. He took the headrope of a creamy-coloured she-camel and swung easily onto her back, whispering the traditional mantra used when mounting a camel: 'Bismillah.' A sharp tap on her ribs with his bare toes, a flourish of his camel stick, and the animal rose, gurgling truculently, to her feet. At a smooth lope, boy and camel disappeared between the dunes. The Bedou looked again at the black camel standing utterly immobile as if carved out of jet. 'Aiwa! Perhaps the Egyptian doctor, Inshallah, can do something. But I doubt it.'

I was in Doha, the capital of Qatar, for a week at the request of Dr Mugahid, Chief of the Qatar Veterinary Services. There were a number of problems to be attended to: a sheik's gazelles in the midst of what might be an epidemic of anthrax, Arabian oryx with skin disease, some ailing falcons inevitably, and a parrot belonging to an important civil servant which apparently had severe glandular trouble. The weather was perfect for tramping about the desert, with opalescent skies, constant light breezes and a still tolerant sun, for it was just before Easter. As well as the wild animals I had been asked to look at a number of domestic ones, doing 'guest appearances' at early morning surgeries at the Central Veterinary Clinic for bemused Bedou who brought goats and sheep for attention. It was like being back in Rochdale all those years before – the same diseases (plus a few bugs that don't exist in the United Kingdom), the same wily smallholders and awkward farmers but transposed from the Pennines to the Gulf and with Lawrence of Arabia costumes instead of clogs and flat caps. I rather enjoyed arguing through the medium of an interpreter with the piquant, colourful characters before going to breakfast with Dr Mugahid on olives, fetta cheese and fresh arab bread.

We were sitting in the air-conditioned pavilion specially built for Her Majesty Queen Elizabeth in order that she might view one of the oryx collections in comfort on the occasion of her state visit to Qatar some years ago, when the message about the black camel reached us. Dr Mugahid is a stocky, warm-humoured ex-academic whose speciality in Egypt had been reproductive physiology. His genial expression changed abruptly to one of grim apprehension on receipt of the news. 'The Ruler's camel, Dr Taylor! We must drive at once to see it.'

It took us a couple of hours through flat and stony desert and then into the dunes to reach the Bedou encampment where the black camel still stood motionless beside the camel keeper's tent. The old Bedou, Mohammed, raised an arm in greeting as we dismounted from the land-cruiser. 'A'salaam aleikum.'

'Aleikum salaam.'

'We trust you are well.'

'Thanks be to God, yes.'

Mugahid introduced me and the camel keeper waved us into the cool interior of his tent. We squatted on a worn Persian carpet that must once have been magnificent, and more formal pleasantries in Arabic were exchanged while other Bedou slipped in and joined us. Mohammed spoke to a young man who went out to return shortly with an elaborate censer made of tin and painted wood. Aromatic smoke poured out of curlicue apertures cut into its top. The camel keeper handed the censer to Dr Mugahid. 'A polite gesture to a visitor,' my colleague explained. 'Incense to sweeten the beard and the body of the weary traveller.' He put the censer under the hem of his loose-hanging shirt and the smoke swirled out round his throat. Then he withdrew it and passed it a few times under his chin, inhaling the fumes appreciatively. 'Now you,' he said, handing me the censer.

I opened the buttons of my shirt and stuck the exotic apparatus with its crackling contents of charcoal and incense against my chest. The blue wreaths of smoke curled about my face and I breathed in the familiar fragrances of High Mass. After me Mohammed and then each of the Bedou used the censer and they all made great play of putting it hard under their chins and fluffing the hairs of their beards in the smoke.

When we were all suitably purified, small cups of cardamom coffee were served while Mohammed explained to Dr Mugahid the problem of the black camel. Formalities concluded, we went outside to examine the patient in question. 'Please, Doctor,' said Mugahid, 'tell us what is wrong with this animal that neither eats nor drinks.'

Mohammed held the headrope while I moved round the

camel, poking and prodding, listening with my stethoscope and peering into its eyes, mouth and nose. Despite not having eaten for many days the camel, true to form, had held on to enough stomach contents, suitably digested, stale and odoriferous, just in case an incense-sweetened veterinarian like me came by. Not for the first time in my life with camels, my stethoscope and I were thoroughly spat upon. A stethoscope is useful not only for listening to hearts and chests but also for picking up the gurgling and squelching sounds of stomach and intestines as they contract. In ruminating animals like camels, the presence of strong, regular contractions of the first stomach, the rumen, is essential. The black camel's innards were silent as the grave – not a gurgle, not a squelch to be heard. But nor could I find any hint of infection. The pulse under the groin (taking which, I nimbly avoided a kick aimed at the same part of my anatomy) was full and regular, and the colour of the gums – scrunch! a warning bite just failed to connect with my shoulder as I ducked – was neither pale nor yellow nor unhealthily red.

I stood back and studied the scene around me. The encampment was in a flat depression perhaps two hundred yards in diameter and entirely surrounded by dunes, wind-honed into the sensuous shapes of the female body. There were three other tents, little more than ragged pieces of sun-bleached canvas on sticks, besides the camel keeper's. The camels and a small herd of black goats just hung around, unrestrained by fence or tether, feeding from piles of hay and lucerne and wooden trays of barley. They were quarrelling, scratching, nibbling, yawning, sleeping and occasionally lusting, but never straying far. The flat ground was littered with the characteristic and ubiquitous debris of the Arabian Gulf countries: 7-Up cans, empty Marlborough cartons, bits of rubber tyre, sheep bones and an assortment of plastic. Among the detritus of modern Arabic civilization in this otherwise romantic spot redolent of Thesiger or Freya Stark, I saw many pieces of plastic string of the sort used to bind hay bales. Lots of stuff around for a bored camel to scoff, I thought – a 7-Up can might be a welcome bouquet garni for a camel on a monotonous diet of hay and barley.

Although atony, a 'going on strike' of the stomach, might be the trouble, I tended more to the idea of something, a foreign body, in the stomach. A plastic bag perhaps? It would have to be a big one, but I'd seen much smaller animals ingest empty fifty-kilo fertiliser bags without any difficulty.

'What do you think?' asked Mugahid as I wiped the bits of green camel spit from my clothes.

'We may have to operate, but first I suggest we try a gentle laxative.'

'Such as?'

'Epsom salts, magnesium sulphate. Get Mohammed to bottle half a kilo into the camel and lots of water. If nothing happens we'd better open the stomach.'

Dr Mugahid looked rather pleased. '*You* will open the stomach, Doctor. How fortunate that you are in Qatar at this time. The Ruler would not want, would not allow the camel to die.'

'But it might. I cannot guarantee . . .'

'Doctor, I am sure you can do it.'

Well, I thought, with any luck the Epsom salts will get things going. And for good measure I'll suggest to Mugahid the use of an injection of carbachol. Operating on a camel that belonged to the Ruler without being quite certain that the stomach was full of rubbish was to be avoided at all costs. 'Epsom salts and carbachol should do something,' I said unconvincingly (at least to myself).

Mugahid went to the land-cruiser and brought the drugs. I stood well back while he injected the carbachol. This time he got spat upon. We drove back to Doha smelling like a travelling sewage works.

I was to be disappointed. The Epsom salts disappeared into the camel's insides and stayed there. Nothing came out. The carbachol produced some copious saliva but no droppings.

The black camel was as depressed and inactive as ever on the next day. The bowels had shut down completely.

'You will have to operate, Doctor,' said Dr Mugahid gleefully. 'It's good to have you here!'

'Mm, yes. I suppose so. Pity about the Epsom salts. You realise that a gastrotomy might not solve the problem? I can't be a hundred per cent certain that there is something in the stomach.' Why couldn't the accursed camel have waited until I'd gone home before falling ill? If anything went wrong I had visions of me making a final appearance in the middle of the main square in Doha after Friday prayers where a big chap with a scimitar would operate on my neck.

The Egyptian smiled expansively and patted my shoulder with a broad hand. 'Like the Omani proverb says, Doctor, "*in kan niyatak 'umar yadurrak darit il-humar*".'

'What's that?'

'It means if your intentions are good, a donkey farting will not hurt you.'

'What I want is to hear that camel farting,' I said.

'In shallah, Doctor, it will – after you do the operation.'

We made plans to operate the following morning as soon as the sun rose. Except in dire emergencies we never give general anaesthetics to animals in tropical countries during the hot periods of the day. Chris, our assistant at Al Ain, gets all his major surgery over by nine o'clock in the morning by the latest.

Doctor Mugahid collected me from my hotel at daybreak and we went first to the Central Veterinary Clinic where a group of his assistants were busy assembling everything we would need to take into the desert. Three land-cruisers would be going, one for Mugahid and me, another for the assistant vets, dressers, technicians and odd-job men – a mixture of Egyptians, Palestinians, Pakistanis, Afghans and Arabs – and a third full of surgical gear and drugs. Gastrotomies on camels under ideal conditions can be done with everything I carry in the Bag and I have done them perfectly satisfactorily with one scalpel, one pair of scissors, one pair of forceps, a needle and

166

some nylon thread in the past, but these conditions were going to be far from ideal. Nevertheless, one would have imagined from all the paraphernalia we had that we were setting out to do at least a heart transplant on an elephant.

About twenty Bedou were waiting for us at the encampment. With our entourage, that made something like three dozen men. Only Mugahid spoke any English. I foresaw problems in keeping the motley gang of helpers and onlookers under control. The first thing, though, was to decide on an operating theatre al fresco. I selected a flat area in the centre of the clearing and signalled to the nearest handful of men to rid it of the 7-Up cans. Although it was still spring, I was glad to see that there were few flies about; on occasion while operating in tropical countries during the cooler season I have watched determined greenbottles actually lay clusters of eggs beside the artery forceps while I worked.

When I had a few square metres of clean sand prepared, I asked Mugahid to tell the camel keeper to bring the black camel over. Slowly, listlessly it walked behind him. Stripped to the waist and ready for another drenching with regurgitated stomach contents (pre-operative scrubbing up can mean something quite special to the camel surgeon!) I injected it in the neck, first with valium and then with xylazine. After a few minutes of gurgling (counting backwards from ten in camelese?), it sank gently to its knees, deeply sedated. So far so good. Now to construct the next phase of my ersatz operating theatre. 'Drive one land-cruiser up along its left side and another along its right. When they are in position, stretch tent material over their roofs from one vehicle to the other. And then fix it with stones.'

Mugahid translated and the men quickly saw the point. A few minutes later the unconscious camel was surrounded by a shaded 'room'. 'Now get two men to hold the material up at one end so that I get enough light.'

With the two men in position as human props, the rest of the people gathered round Mugahid and me as I prepared the

167

operation site itself. I don't think any of the Arab assistant vets had ever seen, let alone done, a camel gastrotomy before, although a couple claimed they had. 'Which side did you operate on?' I asked. 'Left or right flank?'

'Oh, er, right,' they both replied.

I didn't say anything, but opening a camel's right flank would be a disaster – piles of coiled intestines but no stomach anywhere within reach. There's only one way, and that's through the left side. I clipped and shaved the camel's flank about halfway between the last rib and the hip bone. One of the minor skills that a large animal veterinarian should cultivate is the ability to lather and then shave like Sweeney Todd with either a cut-throat razor or a bare safety-razor blade, closely but not too closely. When I first went to university, my father had given me a cut-throat and a patent stropping device, and learning to shave with them (and a styptic pencil) proved very useful in later years.

After the shaving I washed off the flank and disinfected the skin with organic iodine solution. The water I was using came from an open galvanised tank outside the camel keeper's tent but was used by animals and men for all purposes. I washed my hands and arms with mercury soap and then injected a local anaesthetic near the spine to block the nerves supplying the operation site. Satisfied that the deeply dreaming animal wouldn't feel a thing, I draped the shaved area with sterile cloths from an autoclave drum held by Dr Mugahid. I was on my knees, kneecaps already beginning to complain – after years of abuse through kneeling on hard surfaces and exposure to icy water they are beginning to grumble increasingly these days and I can feel sore and gristly nodules on their surfaces. Pressing in close on all sides were our helpers: dark faces, white, yellow and brown teeth, turbans, Arab head-dresses, woolly Afghani caps, Brylcreemed black Pakistani hair, murmurings in Urdu, Pushtu, Arabic and Farsi, the smell of sweat, spices, onions, bad breath and, of course, camel.

168

'Keep back, damn it, give the Doctor some air. Keep out of the light, son of a donkey!' Mugahid railed at them but they took little notice, enthralled as they were by these elaborate rites. I went to great pains to keep my sterile instruments safe in a stainless steel bowl half-filled with iodine solution.

'Tell this fellow to keep away from my hands and arms,' I said to Mugahid as a pair of baggy Afghani pantaloons came close to my fingers.

'Get back, oh addled egg of a scorpion!' shouted Mugahid in Arabic. One of the other men translated the implication into Pushtu for the owner of the pantaloons who didn't speak Arabic. Nonplussed, 'Baggypants' elected to stay put.

'A slip of my scalpel and I'll open his bloody trousers and his leg and cut his balls off!' I bawled. 'Tell him to get back *now*!'

The translators went to work. Baggypants got the message and moved back six inches. A Bedou with a fidgety camel stick immediately took his place and I found him resting a scrawny leg on my left side. Swearing every obscenity I could remember and some that I invented, I began to open the camel's side. Cutting down, I incised skin, muscle and finally the tough peritoneum. Into the opening bulged the glistening wall of the rumen. I fixed the stomach wall to the edges of my incision with four strong clamps and then made a six-inch cut into the interior. I looked down into a black chasm but could see nothing. Foul, warm gases welled out, but my engrossed audience didn't flinch or back an inch.

Carefully I introduced my right hand into the hole. Down it went into the darkness as far as my wrist, and then I felt something hard and round and as big as a grapefruit. It felt like a large, smooth stone. I moved my fingers around and gasped with surprise. More stones, some smaller than the first but some even bigger, filled the stomach cavity. But there was something strange about the stones. So smooth and yet. . . . I went back to the first object I had touched, grasped it and tried to pull it out. But it seemed reluctant to leave its dark cavern and approach the light. As the one stone moved I realised that

169

the others were somehow trying to come along as well. 'I've found the cause of the trouble,' I said to Mugahid. 'Foreign bodies like cannon balls, but for some reason I'm having trouble getting one out.'

Mugahid gave a chortle of delight and told the men what I had said. Immediately to my horror ten, yes ten, brown hands plunged down simultaneously into the operation wound and disappeared alongside mine. The pressure round the stomach incision made it tear at each end and enlarge to accommodate the forest of wrists. My arm was pinned by the men's and there was imminent danger of the clamps losing their grip on the stomach. The open rumen fell back into the abdominal cavity. We would be in a hell of a mess with peritonitis the least of our worries.

'For God's sake, what do they think they're doing? Get out, get out, you idots!' I yelled. 'Get out at once!' But to no avail. The helpers were out of control. My God, were they helping! Babbling excitedly in a babble of tongues, they started to tug at the round stones. Mugahid appeared to have been submerged under a crowd of pushing bodies. I thumped the nearest fellow in the solar plexus with my free hand and luckily connected perfectly. He doubled up, snatching a filthy forearm out of the camel. Now I could get my other arm out. Sterility had gone to the winds. Flailing my arms, I struck out in all directions at the eager instant surgeons and eventually got the operation site clear of human limbs. The clamps luckily had held but the area was heavily contaminated.

Sweating profusely, Mugahid emerged from the mêlée. 'Ignorant devils! Spawn of whores!' he howled. 'How can I apologise for this rabble, Doctor? Is there anything I can do?'

'You just stand between me and them and punch the nose of the first one who gets within a yard of this hole,' I panted. 'I just want to be left alone.'

Slightly dazed, I went back to work. Tidying up the torn stomach incision, I then enlarged it even more and put both hands inside. I grasped the nearest 'stone' and lifted it. Very

170

slowly it came into view – brown and perfectly round and smooth, just like a cannon ball. With great effort I squeezed it out, only to find that it was still attached to something inside the stomach. I slipped a hand past it and felt around. A strong, short cord attached it to the next stone. Gradually I worked that one to the exterior also and again found that it was fixed by yet another cord to a third smooth ball. One by one I brought them out until I had fifty-four 'stones', all linked together by the cords. En masse they would have filled a pair of two-gallon buckets and weighed a total of thirty-two kilos.

When all the strange objects were out, I went in again, checked that the stomach was empty except for a pool of digesting liquid and then began suturing the incision, first the stomach, then the peritoneum and muscle and finally the skin. It was tough work and the effort of pushing the cutting-edged needle through the leathery camel skin lacerated my finger-tips, leaving them painful for days afterwards; despite all the gear, the assistants had neglected to include needle-holders. During the stitching I scattered antibiotic powder liberally into the wound and, when I was satisfied that the camel was securely zipped up, I gave her a massive shot of long-acting tetracycline and some cortico-steroids. God alone knew what those ten arms had introduced into the camel's body cavity.

With the operation completed, I could pay more attention to the strange giant necklace of stones that had been the root of the black camel's illness. I took one of the balls and attacked it with a scalpel. It was as hard as wood. After much effort I managed to cut it in two. It was composed of hair, compressed to a solid mass like rhino horn. The cords were a length of plastic baling twine. Now all could be explained. The twine had been swallowed along with hay or lucerne, an extremely common occurrence, and the hair swallowed over months and years had formed round rough spots or irregularities in the twine much as a pearl grows about a nucleus of a grain of sand. The black camel must have been a great one for licking itself or other camels. Enteroliths (as stones of this kind are called)

171

formed from hair or mineral salts are seen occasionally in other animals. They used to be common in horses in the old days, particularly when much bran was fed. I had seen them before in antelopes and giraffes but never in a camel. And I had never heard of a cluster linked together like grapeshot and of such a combined size.

The assembled company marvelled at the find. No-one could understand how a camel could possibly swallow so many big stones at once. One Bedou apparently explained to another that the strange objects were but a typical cancer. Another claimed I had removed the animal's ovaries and that the black camel would never breed.

After I had washed as well as I could, the camel keeper invited us to his tent for much-needed refreshment. A warm pile of thin pancakes sloppy with almost raw egg and sprinkled with sugar was placed on a tin tray in the middle of the carpet and everyone tore off pieces with their fingers. There was sweet red tea and a huge communal drinking bowl of sour clotted camel's milk. When it was my turn to taste the latter brew I made my excuses and went to check up on the camel. She was waking up. I gave her a light kick on her haunches and she struggled in ungainly fashion to her feet. From her mouth came a subdued but still distinctly choleric and therefore heartening grumble-gurgle. Excellent! Spit on me as much as you like, camel. Just eat and drink and crap again – and live!

Straining my command of Arabic to its limits, I called one of the Bedou camel men. 'Camel. Water,' I said.

He nodded and brought a bucket of water. The black camel drank greedily. 'Alhumdilallah,' said the Bedou as she emptied the bucket.

'Yes, thanks be to God,' I replied. 'Yes indeed.' I went back to the camel keeper's tent and asked Dr Mugahid to arrange for the animal to be given more injections in the next few days and for the operation wound to be cleaned regularly and sprayed with fly repellant.

Now it was time for the formal farewells before leaving.

172

Hands were shaken all round and the ritual words intoned. 'You have brought light to our house.'

'Your house is established.'

'Each and every year.'

'I hope God is bringing us together again.'

'Aye – so be it.'

Mugahid and I walked over to the land-cruiser. 'Do you think she'll be OK now, Doctor?' he asked.

There was no need to reply, we simply gave one another a big Middle Eastern hug, for before I could open my mouth a wonderful, unmistakable and emphatic sound echoed around the rolling dunes. It was the sound of the black camel – farting!

Her flatulent fanfare of farewell did indeed herald her quick recovery. Within twelve hours she was eating again, the wound in her flank healed without complications and two weeks later, when the stitches were removed, she was in the rudest (in every sense) of health.

While I was in Doha, a curious little incident occurred concerning that high-up civil servant's parrot with apparent glandular problems. This miserable and foul-tempered bird, a common Amazon Green which had lost most of its plumage and by rights should have been renamed an Amazon Starkers or Amazon Pink, was apparently the apple of its owner's eye. Even in its bizarre, oven-ready state, due I believe to a hormonal imbalance, he deemed it the finest bird in the world. So the state's veterinary service must forget about all those rare oryx, gazelles, racing camels and such lesser creatures and, on pain of having their soon-to-be-reviewed budget hung, drawn and quartered, get the parrot right. Tariq (the bird had been named after the Moorish conqueror of Spain because the civil servant had purchased him from a bird seller on Las Ramblas De Las Flores in Barcelona) absolutely must be returned to his former befeathered state.

Dr Mugahid had diplomatically explained how very difficult it might be and had drawn the high official's attention to the fact that he himself was bald as an egg. Men have to use toupées, and if medical science can't grow hairs on gentlemen's pates, how could the veterinary service grow feathers on a nude parrot? (Not that Dr Mugahid was suggesting the invention of a patent parrot-feather wig for little Tariq's birthday suit!)

The civil servant had not appreciated the reference to his polished and pristine scalp. 'Birds aren't humans!' he'd snapped with profound insight and considerable asperity. 'Get Tariq's feathers on, Doctor.'

Falconers skilled in the art of 'imping' – replacing broken feathers by sliding a replacement into the shaft of the old one – had been consulted. It was made painfully clear that imping for the parrot was not on. What you can do with the relatively thick quills of a hawk's tail-feathers you haven't a bald parrot in hell's chance of doing all over the chest and pot-belly of the benighted Tariq.

Dr Mugahid's vets had tried the whole range of vitamins as well as powders, sprays, lotions, creams, salves, baths, aerosols, ointments and tinctures. Nothing had grown so much as a millimetre of even the finest down, but all the messing about with him had given the parrot an even more malign temper. He spent his days in a cage in the office of one of Mugahid's young assistants; the civil servant had ordered him 'hospital-ised' until cured. 'Don't send him back till he's as glorious as when I bought him in Spain,' he instructed Mugahid, 'and remember to see your people give him his favourite titbits of pomegranate and pieces of halwa. I want him right for Id-ul-Adha.' The autumn holiday festival was only six months away.

As with the black camel, Dr Mugahid was able to turn responsibility for Tariq over to me during my visit. The civil servant was told that I was in Doha to give an opinion on the mysterious baldness. I didn't mind. Much as I find parrots, especially ones with feather loss or which persistently pluck out their own plumage, difficult to treat, I'd be gone long before Id-ul-Adha. Whereas I have, let us say, a phlegmatic, circumspect affair with the parrot family, Andrew is actually turned on by the little brutes (using the word 'brute' in its precise, unemotive *Oxford English Dictionary* sense meaning 'lower animal') and is actually a member of the Parrot Society, the psittacine equivalent of the Kennel Club in the canine world. Our office at his home in Keighley often has parrot patients of his in for 'R and R' sitting happily in cages on top of filing cabinets or piles of lab reports. I have the sneaking suspicion that Andrew, not to put too fine a point upon it, has a thing about parrots and likes to have them around.

I telephoned my partner and described Tariq and his full-frontal (and posterior) problem. 'Imagine,' I said, 'the parson's nose on an old, plucked boiling fowl – not a pretty sight. This parrot's rear end is like that.'

Typically, Andrew did not prescribe a large dose of barbiturate or a dollop of cyanide into the pomegranate. He even professed hope that the bird might regain its former finery. A series of hormone injections was called for.

Dr Mugahid was cheered up by Andrew's prognostications and so was I, but it seemed to plunge Tariq into an even blacker mood. To give him the first shot into his breast muscle (he reminded me of a partridge ready for marinading in red wine and pine kernels), we needed four people, two to occupy his attention and act as bait for his beak, one to hold him and another to do the actual injecting. He fought like a dervish and managed to take a respectable chunk out of a Pakistani dresser's thumb. Oh, how I love parrots – flitting through the treetops of the Brazilian jungle!

Giving Tariq his injections became the low point of everyone's day at the Central Veterinary Clinic. Cunning folk would be suddenly afflicted with an attack of diarrhoea or devoutly say their prayers when it was time to do battle with the pink peril, others would remember urgent cases at the far side of town and diligently go to attend to them and the majority came to work in leather gloves – rather unusual in the Middle East. One morning I arrived at the clinic to find the place in an uproar. Everyone from Mugahid down to the lowest tea-boy was in a state of hand-wringing consternation. 'What's the matter?' I asked the Chief Vet.

He looked through me with the stare of a man who had had a vision of hell. 'Tariq is gone,' he muttered. 'Gone! Gone!'

'The parrot is dead?' My heart plummeted as the thoughts ran through my mind: Civil servant told parrot is dead. How did it happen? Injections as ordered by the doctor from England. Right, out to the desert with the swine! Bury him up to his eyeballs in an ant-hill!

'No, he is not dead.' Mugahid's words snapped back my attention. 'Just gone. Escaped.'

'Escaped? How?' Tariq as an escapee was almost as bad news as Tariq the late and unlamented.

'We don't know, Doctor. We have searched everywhere, in the assistant's room where he was, in the clinic, in the garden, everywhere. I even have two men scouring the streets nearby. Not a sign of him.'

'But a naked bird like that couldn't fly far, if at all.' Then I imagined the rheumy-eyed and preposterous figure of Tariq, looking rather like a minute Colonel Blimp fresh from the Turkish bath and marching cussedly through the desert.

'Maybe he has been kidnapped or killed,' Mugahid suggested.

'Possible. Plenty of folk here hate his guts. Doctor, do you think the Pakistani with the bitten thumb. . . ?'

'No, I've interrogated him thoroughly.' Doctor Mugahid sat hopelessly on the corner of his desk. 'I'm not sure how you say it in English,' he sighed, 'but translating from the Arabic, you and me are like two cats blindly chasing a fly that has settled on the surface of a cesspool.'

'I know what you mean. We are in the sewage if we don't find that parrot.'

'Exactly.'

'Come on let's begin a completely new search all over again. We'll start with his cage.'

The assistant vet's room was small and austere. It contained a desk, a chair and a filing cabinet – nothing else, apart from the empty parrot cage which stood on the floor by the desk with its door open. Parrots are rather good at undoing latches. I looked at the cage carefully. A character like Tariq would have had little difficulty with the simple clip lock. There was nowhere the parrot could hide in the room, so next I turned to the door of the room itself. It was a wooden frame filled with intact mosquito-proof wire and it closed automatically by means of a strong spring. Opening the door against the spring needed considerable pressure – more than a parrot could exert – and, when released, it closed quickly. The door couldn't have been accidentally left ajar, so either Tariq, having escaped from his cage, positioned himself by the door and nipped out smartly when someone came in, or he was indeed kidnapped.

'Why would someone take him?' Mugahid asked. Why indeed? People needed Tariq like a hole in the head – except of course for his doting owner.

'For ransom?' I suggested. It was surrealistic, a fantasy. A phone call to the civil servant: 'Listen carefully, I'll only say it once. Half a million ryals to be left in a bag next to the fourth camel on the left down the road to Saudi. Otherwise, it's curtains for your parrot. Listen, he's squawking into the phone to prove he's still alive. But he won't be for long. Pay up by tomorrow night or you'll get one of his claws in the post!' No – I couldn't imagine anybody kidnapping Tariq, but it might be worth asking the police to check whether the hospitals had admitted any patients with amputated fingers within the past twenty-four hours.

We conducted the new search in a logical manner. Every office, laboratory, surgery, loosebox and store room was thoroughly combed. Then we scoured every inch of the gardens. No parrot. The men who had been out in the streets came back empty-handed and crestfallen. Tariq had apparently vanished without trace. I couldn't get over the obvious fact that the almost featherless bird (and those plumes which remained were only on his head) would have been incapable of flying. A frenzied flutter maybe, but no lift-off. If he had gone AWOL it must have been by legging it. But parrots with their awkward, side-to-side-rocking gait aren't roadrunners or ostriches and Tariq would be lucky if he could clock up more than half a mile an hour. And then there was the problem of the spring-loaded door to the room in which he had been hospitalised. He couldn't possibly have opened that himself.

I went into the room again and stood pondering. Desk, chair, filing cabinet. The filing cabinet was of a common design, made in metal and with three large drawers tightly closed. I pulled open the top drawer: racks of papers in cardboard folders. Not enough room for a sparrow, let alone a parrot. I opened the middle drawer: more documents, rank after rank. Parrots can't get into closed filing cabinets, I told myself, but nevertheless I pulled out the bottom drawer. It again was full of green folders. Just as I was about to slam it shut, I caught a glimpse of something pink among the green. Nestling down between two bulging files and glaring at me with a look fit to kill was Tariq. I stood and stared. Suddenly the parrot reached up with his beak and grasped one of the runners on which the drawer was suspended. Arching his neck, eyes bulging with the effort, claws dug into the file in front of him, he started to haul the drawer shut. Slowly, smoothly it began to close. I could hear his beak clicking against the metal each time he changed his hold. Clunk! The drawer was shut. Tariq had withdrawn into his ingenious sanctum sanctorum.

Ignominiously hauled out and restored to his cage, Tariq cursed all and sundry in the most frightful way. The staff of the clinic cheered when they heard of the absconder's apprehension, and much sweet tea and 7-Up was drunk in celebration. A piece of wire was fastened round the catch on the door of the parrot's cage. That should have fixed him, but next day Tariq had disappeared again. The wire on the catch had been bitten through and the filing cabinet drawers were all as they should be – neatly shut. Dr Mugahid and I smiled as I opened the bottom drawer. 'Out you come,' I said as the racks of files slid out. But this time there was no parrot among the postmortem reports and reprints of scientific articles. We found him in the top drawer, crouched behind the last sheaf of documents, beak within easy reach of the right-hand runner. Again, as soon as I released my grip on the drawer handle, he pulled the files and himself back into the darkness and probably hoped we'd go away. Tariq must have been as adept at climbing up the cabinet and pulling the drawers open as he was at shutting them.

With Tariq back in his cage yet again, we secured it with a bicycle padlock. He never did a bunk again, at least not during the rest of his stay at the clinic. I received a letter from Dr Mugahid when the Id festival came round. He sent me his greetings and informed me that Tariq was indeed once more a fully fledged Amazon Green. His owner, the civil servant, had taken him home in delight, but the budget for the Central Veterinary Clinic had still been slashed by a vicious thirty per cent. Tariq, the parrot with friends in high places, can maybe pull strings as well as filing cabinet runners!

10   A Life in the Day of . . .

'They're turning bright pink and dying by the dozen! Can you please ring as soon as possible?' The radio telephone operator couldn't disguise the alarm in her normally cool and professional voice. I used the same channel on my mobile radio when travelling round Britain by car as some of the emergency medical services and, although the operator was accustomed to handling babies turning blue, miscarriages and all manner of other human dramas, this sounded to her like the beginning of Armageddon. I pressed the answer button on my microphone as the car turned into Byfleet and joined the sluggish stream of commuting traffic moving towards Weybridge.

'What is turning pink exactly? Over.'

'Er sorry, Ebony 314, I don't know. The message has been passed through Manchester and Reading Air Calls. All I've got is that and the place. Anything else must have got lost in transmission.'

The place from which the message had come – the Welsh Mountain Zoo at Colwyn Bay – was the key thing and the reason I didn't break out into a cold sweat at the news of multiple deaths from some sort of mysterious pink plague. I was pretty certain as to the species of animal involved. 'Roger. I'll attend to it as soon as possible. Ebony 314 standing by.'

The Welsh Mountain Zoo, a delightful park set on top of a hill with magnificent vistas over the North Wales countryside and coastline, has elephants, lions and monkeys like other zoos and breeds sea-lions and provides bird of prey displays better than most. It also has a locust breeding unit. These fascinating insects make a valuable wholefood addition to the diets of many birds and mammals and the Welsh Mountain Zoo is so successful at farming locusts that they are able to supply them to other zoos and bird gardens all over the country.

Locusts are the only true insects that I've ever had to treat for disease. They are also the only insects I have ever eaten – after frying them like chips on an 'Animal Magic' programme. At Belle Vue I'd taken a keen interest in rearing them and had presented the zoo with a metal and glass breeding unit which had functioned well enough to keep most of the insectivorous animals happily victualled. Simple to feed on greens and cereals, they do demand careful control of their environment and high standards of hygiene in order to avoid worm infestations, diarrhoea and attacks by microbes. When a locust's normal colours of green, yellow and black change to a rather shocking pink and they begin to die, it is usually due to infection with a particular bacterium. At the next phone box I would ring Nick Jackson at the Welsh Mountain Zoo and discuss moving the surviving locusts to a clean unit and spraying the daily ration of cut grass with a suitable antibiotic dissolved in water.

A radio telephone in the car had played a vital part in saving a number of animals' lives over the years, and before Andrew joined me it had been even more essential. Nevertheless, from time to time, because of the nature of the system which did not allow direct communication but went via an operator, there were mangled messages to unravel as I rushed along the motorways or ground my way through London in the middle of the day. Sometimes an operator just couldn't believe that the message she was passing wasn't a joke: 'I've got a nutter here who says he's got a constipated gorilla!' or 'A foreign-sounding person keeps calling you about a whale with influenza. Do you think one of your friends is fooling around, Dr Taylor?' No, no-one was ever fooling around.

When Clyde, the veteran performing dolphin now at

Woburn, was at the London Dolphinarium in 1971, he fell ill with severe hepatitis. I was still based in the North and travelled frequently down to London to supervise his treatment, on one occasion going twice from Rochdale to London and back in a single day and picking up two speeding convictions en route. As the days of multiple injections and force-feeding passed by, we watched anxiously for the first signs of an improvement in Clyde's condition. Would some liver cells remain functioning long enough for their amazing powers of multiplication and recuperation to come into play? The prognosis was bad: most hepatitis cases in dolphins at that time ended fatally. One evening, after visiting the thin and depressed animal bobbing up and down feebly in his holding pool and after taking yet another blood sample for monitoring of liver enzymes, I was driving back up the M1 when the radio telephone operator came on the air with my call sign. She had a message from the London Dolphinarium. Gary Marshall, the trainer doing the night watch, staying by Clyde's pool in a sleeping bag, was on the phone. My heart sank. It could only mean one thing: Clyde's liver had lost the battle. I would have to turn round at the next exit and go back to arrange the autopsy.

'Ebony 314. Mr Marshall says . . .' she hesitated. 'Clyde's tool is out. Over.'

'Say again, please. Over.'

'Clyde's tool is out. Over.'

I was nonplussed. Garbled message, undoubtedly. Clyde has passed out? Clyde's been taken out? It must mean something like that. 'Say again, please,' I repeated. 'I don't understand.'

There was perhaps thirty seconds silence. Then the girl's voice began again. 'Ebony 314. Clyde's tool is out.'

Still nonplussed, I pressed the button once more. 'Please say yet again and spell second word.'

'Clyde's tool is out. T-o-o-l. Tool!'

Suddenly the penny dropped and I realised what Gary meant. Feeling myself actually blush at the undoubted embarrassment I had caused the operator, I hurriedly acknowledged the message and went off the air. And I felt utterly elated!

What Gary had quite rightly wanted to tell me was very good news indeed. Clyde was swimming around his pool with unmistakable signs of sexual arousal. He must be feeling better! Not quite sure how to put it in case the operator would at best take it as a joke in poor taste or at worst phone the police to deal with an obscene caller, he had decided to use one of the mildest pseudonyms for the male phallus and one which with any luck the lady operator might not associate at all with genitalia. 'Clyde's tool is out' could conceivably be a reference to, say, shipbuilding or engineering. As Gary explained to me later, 'Clyde's tool is out' might be the headline announcing that a famous Scottish firm had got a strike problem, though why anyone should think a zoo vet half way up the M1 would want to hear the latest on industrial relations at a quarter to midnight is another matter!

The following day I phoned Air Call to explain the position to the operator. I needn't have worried. When I told her how Clyde had turned the corner and looked like making it she said, 'Marvellous, Doctor. Just what me and the girls said when the call came in. Not much wrong with Clyde, whoever or whatever he is, if he's feeling his oats like that!'

Bright girls, the Air Call girls. And they were right. Clyde never looked back after playing Priapus that night. His liver healed and, if he dies of anything, I'm sure it will be of old age.

That man in the pub, or that lady in the post office, often say, 'Must be a great job, yours. Want someone to carry your bag?' It is paradoxically the best and the worst job in the world, and for me it has meant exquisite pleasure, deepest depression and a divorce. The vet in a suitcase, hopping from zoo to safari park to marineland around the world, lives a life of great loneliness. Friends everywhere but almost always isolated. Home, colleagues in the profession (what profession – zoo vets have little in common with farm and small animal vets): they exist, but somewhere else. The social life is excellent while working, but at home the tyrant telephone can and generally does destroy holidays, dinner parties and weekend lie-ins. I have spent four Christmasses and five New Years away from home, screwed up maybe twenty holidays, broken a hundred speaking engagements and missed a thousand meals with friends.

And yet, and yet, I cannot bring myself to write that I regret it. Although I sometimes feel that every exotic patient I touch takes the pressure of my fingers as a valediction and permission to die, there are the good, the great, the ecstatic times – when a Clyde comes through or a penguin chick with rickets straightens his back and at last puts on his adult plumage or a crocodile who hasn't eaten for a year snaps at a proffered chunk of beef. Zoo vets, and I see this in Andrew too very plainly, are like junkies: once hooked on the problems of everything from aardvark to zebra, they are addicted more intensely than those who crave heroine. I could never return to the world of cats and cattle of pigs and puppies. Porcupines and pumas get into the blood.

Often I am asked what I do on a normal day. A normal day? What is that? At home in Lightwater the day begins when the first phone call arouses me from sleep. It may be Antibes one hour, Tel Aviv three hours, the Gulf four hours or Hong Kong eight hours ahead. Whatever it is, it's not small talk. Something is in trouble. When I put the receiver down I go and make tea for Hanne and myself and then, still in my pyjamas, go through the mail. A photograph of a strange skin lesion on a sea-lion in New Zealand, a dolphin trainer in Germany who requests a reference, a sample of pus from a wallaby with boils in Spain for analysis, a lady in Saffron Walden who has arthritis and wants me to use acupuncture on her legs like I did with a giraffe, the lab results on the latest blood sample of the Windsor whale, an invitation to speak to the Bagshot Wolf Cubs on 'Animals I Have Known', bills from the drug companies, airlines, American Express, Diners Club etc, and a strange missive from an animal liberationist who thinks I'm a monster in working for captive animals – the signature is smeared with human excrement.

Washed and dressed, I discuss the hypothetical outline of my day with Hanne over an egg and two pieces of toast (she watches my weight carefully). The phone really starts getting agitated by 8.30 am. A Baptist Minister in Wales is looking for a German acquaintance who claimed to have been a veterinarian specialising in brain surgery in rhinos. He's lost touch with him. I tell him his acquaintance must be odd, to say the least: there are no specialists in rhino brain surgery. No-one has ever opened a living rhino's skull.

Next, Andrew phones to say he's at Gatwick about to leave for Houston, Texas. We discuss a tricky case of a buffalo with thyroid disease and arrange to telex the owner. Nine o'clock and I'm on the road to Weybridge to do the weekly inspection of Gordon Mills' private collection of apes. Mills is Tom Jones' and many other stars' agent. In the garden of his luxurious Surrey home he has a primate unit finer than most zoos' and looked after by one of the most brilliant ape keepers in Europe, Jeremy Keeling. What I like about the Mills collection is the opportunity to meet two very old and good friends: Jane, the female orang from Belle Vue whom my ex-wife, Shelagh, nursed through post-natal depression,* and Louie, the male orang who used to be at Flamingo Park when I was Veterinary Officer there. And Gordon Mills' gorillas are magnificent creatures!

Jeremy and I talk about the finer points of ape management for half an hour or so and then I go on to Chessington – the young beavers there need sexing. After Chessington I take the A3 to London and make my way to the library of the Royal College of Veterinary Surgeons to do some reading on the effect of isoniazid on cats. I've got to give an opinion in a case in Italy where a vet gave the drug to a bunch of cheetahs which he suspected had TB and killed the lot. In the library I meet my teacher of medicine of long ago, Professor McIntyre, and we

*See *Doctor in the Zoo*.

nip off for a coffee together. My pocket bleeper disturbs the peace of the RCVS library when we return, and I phone in to hear that there are problems in Madrid. A call to Iberia and I am on my way home. My mood declining, I slip a Vivaldi cassette into the slot of the player.

Hanne has my bag packed, a French bread pizza heated and a beer in the glass by the time I arrive, and while I eat takes notes of things which I should have done but now can't. She'll go to dinner at The Pantiles tonight with Andreas, her elder son, instead of me. At Heathrow David Bellamy rushes up, pounds my hand and asks me to be sure to write to someone about the terrible things they're doing to the Barrier Reef ecology in Australia, then disappears into the crowd. I phone Hanne as usual from the airport. 'Contact Tel Aviv at once,' she tells me. 'They need advice about a sick sea-lion before you board.' I get through to Israel, discuss the trouble with the local vet, Eli Kutin, and then dash for the plane.

During the flight I write what you, dear reader, are now inwardly digesting. There's two hours – enough for a couple of gin and tonics and three thousand words. At Barajas Airport, Madrid, the customs officer asks why I am carrying so many drugs. I use the magic phrase, 'Para los animales del rey' – for the King's animals – and as always go through like the wind. No-one to meet me this time, so I take a taxi to the zoo. The taxi driver wants to talk about football, but I can understand only half of his Spanish and even less of his obviously encyclopedic knowledge of English football.

At the zoo in the Casa de Campo I am on 'home ground'. Antonio-Luis and Liliana, my best of friends, make coffee and explain the current problems: an anaemic baby chimpanzee brought in illegally from Guinea, confiscated and now in quarantine at the zoo; and a female eland antelope with a prolapsed vagina and bladder. I go to pay my respects to the zoo financial director and the zoo biological director and then set to work. The chimpanzee needs a transfusion. We take blood from another chimp with the same group (A plus) and drip it into the tranquillised baby. It looks pretty bad to me – there are signs of mental disability as well. Then on to the eland. Antonio-Luis darts it by blow pipe with Immobilon and I do the operation. Emptying the prolapsed bladder, I replace everything into the pelvis and then put a sterilised plastic milk bottle into the vagina to hold it. I stitch the milk bottle to the vulva, using sterilised, plastic-coated electric cable, and spread the pressure by means of broad plastic tubing.

It is ten o'clock by the time we are finished. The three of us go to a *tapas* bar for beer, octopus and anchovies in vinegar. My knee caps are aching again; it's that kneeling in icy water in Iceland. Into my friends' battered old Citroën and we drive out to their apartment where I have a permanent bedroom. There's a message on their answering machine from Holland: would I please ring as soon as possible about a hippopotamus with a cough. I make the call, prescribe Bisolvon and then take coffee and Carlos Primero before going to bed. We talk about how troublesome giraffes are to anaesthetise. By 11.30 I'm in bed.

At midnight Liliana wakes me. Andrew is calling from the USA – could I please go to Denmark tomorrow. Asleep again, I dream of dolphins in operating gowns and elephants holding syringes in their trunks with which they inject my buttocks. Hanne phones at 1 am – the sea lion in Tel Aviv has just gone into a coma. And that's the end of my 'normal' day.

'What's your favourite animal?' is the next most common question I am asked. It is not easy, perhaps impossible, to answer. Of course Chu-Lin, the baby panda, the dolphin, the orang-utan, the elephant, but then there's also the Vietnamese pot-bellied pig, the takin, the colobus monkey. And certainly all the stray moggies who have over the years adopted us – Buck-tooth, Tom, Lupin, Lenin and the rest, the very best of companions. So perhaps it would be easier to approach the question from the opposite direction and ask which animals aren't my favourites. Parrots perhaps, horses, greyhounds.

No, if I were to be really honest I think I must say that my favourites are the frogs (and their cousins the toads). Your ordinary common or garden frog turns me on. The magic of spring days going a-tadpoling when I was a boy still persists and, when I travel to Switzerland now to see my friends Conny and Gerda Gasser at their marineland in Lipperswil, I get a great kick out of seeing that the road sign near their home, a big red triangle enclosing a black frog upon a white ground, signifying 'Caution – frogs crossing', is well maintained, its paint sparkling and fresh, by the worthy local Cantonal authorities. When the Swiss (or British) frogs go courting en masse, they are blind to the highway code as they cross roads to reach the breeding waters. Just as hedgehogs so desperately deserve the cattle-grid escape routes that they are now being provided with in enlightened parts of the country, so frogs should have right of way over human beings who drive like Mr Toad.

Sadly, I am virtually never called upon to treat sick frogs. When pesticides killed the wondrous giant Goliath frogs, brought at great expense and risk to human health from the night-time jungles of Spanish Guinea to Duisburg Zoo in Germany, there was nothing we could do. In the past ten years I have had but one amphibian patient – a marine toad, one of the comical creatures that sit, each under his very own adopted village lamp-post in South America, catching flies and moths attracted by the light after nightfall. This fellow, with a Falstaffian paunch and a strong facial resemblance to Sir Robin Day, had contracted tuberculosis of the eyelids. Tiny amounts of rifampicin, mixed with the tinned dog food that he avidly scoffed, cleared the infection after about four months treatment. His owner, a lady hairdresser in Richmond, who kept him in her sauna and never took holidays because she didn't trust anyone to take care of 'Buggerlugs' (yes, that really was his name) while she was away, paid my fee by barter and I got half a dozen shampoo, trim and sets with manicure in her unisex salon. I have never been so well groomed, before or since, as when I treated Buggerlugs.

The most exquisite of frogs are the tree and arrow frogs of South America. Tiny, fragile, difficult-to-maintain creatures, they are gorgeous in their brilliant coloured skins of red, green, blue and yellow. The best and the most successful exhibition of tree frogs that I know is at Ouwehands Zoo in Holland. There, brilliant purple and yellow tree frogs from Surinam live in a perfectly constructed natural habitat amongst dripping rocks, caves, moss, toadstools, ferns and still pools, and feed upon a specially bred mutation of fruit flies that don't grow wings and fly unco-operatively away. Throw in a pinch of these insects and the little frogs hop about gleefully, gobbling up their tasty titbits. A joy to watch!

In 1982 a singular incident occured at Al Ain, concerning red arrow frogs. Peter Dickinson, one of the curators and a specialist reptile and amphibian man, set up a fine vivarium for a group of these little animals. It is a well-known fact that the Indians of the South American jungle have traditionally used arrow frogs for help in hunting. Cruelly impaling them on twigs, they roast them slowly over a fire and collect the drops of liquid which exude from the frog's skin. This juice is a deadly, curare-like toxin and, applied to the points of blow pipe darts and hunting arrows, quickly kills birds and mammals, even as big as jaguars. Its effects on humans if struck by one of the treated missiles is also likely to be lethal. For years I had on occasion, out of pure interest and delight, handled arrow frogs in zoos up and down Europe. I'd never dream of roasting one and no-one so far had ever jabbed me in the backside with a poisoned Amerindian arrow. There seemed to be no reason for avoiding contact between one's hand and an unroasted, living and apparently friendly arrow frog.

Peter received the consignment of arrow frogs, efficiently packed in plastic boxes, one to a box with bedding of damp cotton wool and plastic foam glued to the underside of the lids to prevent the frogs getting headaches if they did a bit of hopping around en route. He at once unpacked them and with

189

his fingers carefully placed each tiny scarlet amphibian into the ersatz jungle that he had created.

Two minutes after handling the last frog, Peter began to feel rather odd. His heart was banging in a peculiar way and his chest became tight. Soon breathing was difficult. The curator sat on the floor in the reptile house, wondering vaguely if he was having a heart attack and waiting for one of his staff to come by and send for help. But on-one came, and Chris Furley and I in the veterinary clinic a stone's throw away were totally unaware of Peter's plight. After about thirty minutes during which he had the feeling that his body, totally numb, was separating from his head, be began to breathe a little easier and the weakness started to recede. Eventually he managed to get to his feet and totter out and make his way to our clinic. Thereafter Peter's recovery was rapid. A strong cup of Chris's tea and a cigarette, and within an hour he was back to normal.

I have no doubt that the curator was poisoned by arrow frog toxins merely by touching them, something I had never come across before. His hands, which we inspected, bore nothing more than the odd minute abrasions which one would expect in a man living an essentially outdoor life in a desert zoo, but through one of these almost invisible breaks in the skin surface enough of the moisture from the frogs' skins, fortunately in a sub-lethal dose, had been able to pass to produce distinct signs of poisoning. In future I would handle such pretty little animals with even greater respect (and rubber gloves). Their startling colours are meant as a warning – hands off!

As you might expect, danger lurks in a zoo in a variety of guises besides that of the winsome, wide-eyed and minuscule arrow frogs. There is no question that the big cats pose the greatest physical threat to staff and visitors. Each year a handful of people are killed by tigers and lions in European safari parks, circuses and, to a lesser extent, zoos. It isn't just the foolish tourist who, ignoring all the warning notices, opens his car window for a close-up snapshot or the guy with the puncture in the lion reserve who, instead of honking his horn to draw the attention of the wardens, sends his eight-year-old daughter to run and tell them – this actually happened in a Spanish safari park in 1982. As he said to the police later, 'I thought she was a better runner than me.' She probably was, but she couldn't match the speed of four adult lionesses. It isn't just the mentally disturbed like the religious maniac at Rio Leon Safari Park in Spain who wanted to 'speak peace to the wild beasts'. Twice he was caught climbing semi-naked over the fence into the big cat reserve. The third time he managed it, unobserved by the keepers, and walked open-armed towards a pride of lions 'speaking peace'. The lions, as opposed to unilateralism as Margaret Thatcher is, promptly ate him.

No, the professionals, the zoo men often with years of experience in handling dangerous beasts, also fall victim with monotonous regularity. I have lost a number of good friends, keen big cat keepers, who made one tiny slip, dropped their guard for a fraction of a second, become over-confident or complacent with animals they had reared from cubs. Or they too often tried to take liberties with animals which do not think in the way humans do, with which we cannot communicate, whose behaviour we only partially understand and which, particularly in the case of the tiger, are frighteningly fast on their feet. Tigers combine surprise, phenomenal acceleration and a heavy body to launch an attack. Unlike polar bears, which are southpaws and only ever use their right paw for attack or defence, tigers punch equally well with both paws; a single clubbing blow will fell any man and then it is a simple matter for the cat to deliver its favourite, instinctive coup de grâce – a neat bite to the neck which severs the spinal cord. In this manner keepers have been killed in recent years at Windsor, John Aspinall's zoo in Kent (two men within a month of one another and by the same tigress when she was separated from her cub at cleaning time), at Hodenhagen in Germany and at several other places.

At Hodenhagen, Simon Compton-Hall, an English keeper whom I knew well, had struck up what he believed to be a cast-iron relationship with thirteen big Bengal tigers (unlucky number). Two days after I had visited the park and discussed with him our management of a unique epidemic of brain disease in the big cats which so far has affected only Hodenhagen and certain other West German safari parks, Simon walked among the thirteen tigers and persuaded one animal to stand on its hind legs and place its forepaws against a 'Stay inside your car' placard as if reading it, so that a local newspaper man could take photographs. As my friend arranged the tiger's limbs, another tiger, feeling left out of things, jealously tapped him on the back of the leg much in the way that your fireside cat draws your attention to himself. But a tap from a tabby is nothing, whereas a tap from a tiger buckles your knees for sure. Simon fell to the ground while still holding the first tiger's forelegs. Startled by the keeper's sudden movement and a tug on its legs, this animal reverted automatically to type, to the lone jungle hunter that must react by instant reflex to the unusual and unexpected, to the killer machine. As Simon lay on the ground the first tiger began to maul him, its excitement affected the second and, like a nuclear chain reaction, then spread to the other eleven animals. The entire group moved in. Mercifully Simon died quickly, his end recorded by the newspaper man who despicably filmed every detail instead of driving his car, in which he safely sat, at the tigers and scattering them. The photographs were published in newspapers and periodicals all over the world and no doubt brought the man a great deal of money. I wonder if he sleeps easily with the memory of his cowardice and macabre opportunism.

For myself, when working with such animals there is no room for bravado or chance-taking. One bite from an alsatian isn't going to kill a vet. One bite from a tiger is likely to be curtains. With the restraint cages, tranquillisers, sedatives, blow pipes, pole syringes and long-range dart guns at our disposal nowadays, there is no need to take risks. Last year I visited an awful, run-down (and in parts completely inhumane) safari park in Spain, El Rincon. Liliana was with me to make an evaluation of the place for a company which had recently purchased it. The head keeper, a grizzled Spaniard in his fifties, took us round in a battered Volkswagen with his window, I noticed, wide open. When we entered the tiger section I drew the window to his attention. 'Do you not think that you should close the window?' I said.

'Why?'

'Because of the tigers. '

The Spaniard laughed and patted my shoulder. 'Don' worry Doctor, don' worry. Anyway the window won't close. There's no glass in the door.'

'Tigers are too dangerous, Señor, for cars with no glass in their doors.'

He laughed patronisingly again. 'Doctor, are you scared of big pussy cats or something? I thought you had been around zoos a bit. Thought you were a big guy, thought you weren't scared of big pussy cats.'

'Amigo, I have been round zoos a long time. I do know a lot about tigers. I am scared of them. Very scared.'

The head keeper grinned, whistled and pulled a long face. 'Me,' he said, waving a hand airily out of the window, 'me I'm not scared of nothing. Don' need no window. I got these tigers under control.'

'How long have you been working here?'

'Six months, more or less.'

'And before that?'

'Worked on a farm, Doctor. Not scared of nothing!' He gave me a pitying look and I gave him about three months if he carried on like that. One day for sure a tiger would stalk his car and pull him out of that open window by his scalp before you could say 'Viva España'.

'If he's head keeper with just half a year's experience of exotic animals, what must his keepers be like?' remarked Liliana as we drove away. When later we made our report to the company, we recommended that the head keeper be fired immediately. To save his life.

My greatest fear among the inmates of a zoological collection is reserved for the venomous snakes. Handling them is always perilous. If there is any misunderstanding or less than total co-ordination between me and the reptile keeper who holds the snake while I pass a stomach tube, paint areas of mouth rot with streptomycin solution or inject an anti-worm preparation, a toxic bite can be inflicted in a flash. To slow down dangerous specimens before treatment, I arrange if possible for the temperature in their vivaria to be turned down. The colder environment makes them more sluggish and, I hope, not quite so fast with their fangs. But I'm always relieved when the animal is back in its quarters and the door is shut tight behind it. Of course all serpentaria possessing venomous species have vials of antiserum in the fridge to be rushed to the hospital along with any bitten person, but the antiserum for certain species can produce more damage in the human body than the bite itself. Treatment of snake bite needs a lot of specialised knowledge on the part of the doctors involved. It isn't just a question of jabbing the victim with the appropriate antiserum. Unfortunately, and understandably, doctors in Great Britain have generally no experience of the effects of mamba, rattlesnake, krait and gaboon viper. Even in Al Ain, where there are local poisonous snakes, Chris Furley has to be called in to advise when the hospital receives a case of snake bite.

If you must get bitten by a cobra or a tiger snake in England, try to arrange for it to be done in the Liverpool or London areas, as only in these cities are there specialists who can give you more than a fighting chance. Luckily the tendency nowadays is for more and more zoos to keep only non-venomous reptiles. One last tip: temperance pays in the reptile house. The bite of the only poisonous lizards in the world, the gila monster and the beaded lizard, have so far proved fatal only in drunks!

There are many other less deadly but still potentially

194

dangerous beasts in the zoo – camels, zebras, giraffes and certain antelopes among them. When I was making a 'World About Us' film at Windsor some years ago, a bold giraffe walked up to me quietly and then gratuitously threw a foreleg kick at my head which would have brained me if I hadn't ducked in the nick of time. It's all on film! I was at a Dutch zoo when the eland keeper, an old and experienced man who knew his antelopes as well as a shepherd knows his sheep, was suddenly and for no apparent reason attacked by one of his charges as he was releasing them from their night houses. The eland's horns passed straight through his body and he died quickly in the most horrific way as the animal carried him, impaled, with its head held high, out to the paddock.

There are other dangers. Exotic animals can carry exotic as well as more commonplace diseases, and some of them can be a serious health hazard for human beings, particularly where a zoo has a quarantine section receiving newly imported stock. Strict governmental control is exercised over potential carriers of rabies and other dread virus infections such as Marburg disease and B-virus. Marburg disease suddenly appeared out of nowhere in the mid-1960s and was transmitted to humans by African monkeys. Everyone who contracted the infection died. B-virus similarly kills most human victims and leaves a few with permanent central nervous system damage; in monkeys, however, it causes nothing more than a mild bleb on the lips identical to a human 'cold sore'. It's no joke doing quarantine inspection as a veterinary surgeon and finding a monkey with a small mark or blister in the mouth region. It might be a simple abrasion or an unimportant bacterial infection, but it might also be the B-virus. At such moments, luckily rare, I cross my fingers and pray that my gown, mask, goggles, rubber gloves and wellington boots will do their stuff and keep me inviolate. The shower and povidone antiseptic lather from tip to toe can't come quickly enough.

In some countries such as Spain there is a fairly high incidence of tuberculosis both among the human population and in zoo animals. The infection can travel both ways and it is as important for us to arrange screening of all zoo personnel to avoid them infecting animals as it is to do skin, blood and bateriological tests on the animals to prevent them passing TB to visitors and staff. It is fortunate that tuberculosis in humans and, where advisable, in animals can now be so successfully treated.

Parrot disease, psittacosis, is another risk to the zoo vet, but Andrew and I have been very lucky over the years. Despite all the bugs we have undoubtedly encountered in examining countless infected creatures all over the world, in the wild, in quarantine and in zoos proper, and after thousands of autopsies, some conducted in far from ideal conditions without running water, good light or adequate protective clothing, we have with one exception never had the slightest occupational disease. No ringworm from lions, no erysipeloid from dolphins, no shigellosis from monkeys, no hepatitis from chimpanzees, no lung fungus from penguins. Maybe it's the little pen sprays of undertaker's antiseptic liquid soap that we carry for emergency use in the field. Then in 1982 Andrew, just back from the Middle East where he'd inspected birds arriving from Africa, went down with a severe super-flu that for the first time in our partnership stopped him working for weeks and was eventually diagnosed as psittacosis. I always knew Andrew's love-affair with parrots was bound to end in tears! Touch wood, the parrots haven't got me yet.